Medical
Philosophy

Conceptual Issues
in Medicine

Medical Philosophy

Conceptual Issues
in Medicine

Mario Bunge
McGill University, Canada

by

ientific Publishing Co. Pte. Ltd.
ck Link, Singapore 596224
e: 27 Warren Street, Suite 401-402, Hackensack, NJ 07601
: 57 Shelton Street, Covent Garden, London WC2H 9HE

of Congress Cataloging-in-Publication Data
lario, 1919–
al philosophy : conceptual issues in medicine / Mario Bunge.
m.
es bibliographical references and index.
978-9814508940 (softcover : alk. paper)

: 1. Philosophy, Medical. W 61]

dc23
                            2013008779

ibrary Cataloguing-in-Publication Data
ue record for this book is available from the British Library.

am Osler at the bedside: inspection, palpation, auscultation, contemplation.
chael Bliss' *William Osler: A Life in Medicine* (University of Toronto Press, 1999).

ernard (1813–1878).
e *Popular Science Monthly*, Vol. 13, 1878.

Editor: Veronica Low

oy Stallion Press
nquiries@stallionpress.com

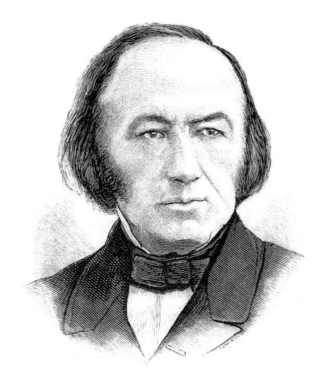

Claude Bernard (1813–1878), the father of experimental medicine
and an eminent philosopher of science.

PREFACE

Several current controversies in the medical community are about key concepts or comprehensive assumptions. Hence, they are actually philosophical rather than medical, even though they are often discussed in the *Lancet, New England Journal of Medicine,* and *British Medical Journal.* Let this short list of questions suffice to prove the existence of iatrophilosophy, or the philosophy of medicine: whether a disease is just a cluster of signs or biomarkers of it; whether a bunch of clinical data suffices to describe a disease and make a correct diagnosis; whether contemporary medicine is peculiar in being evidence-based; whether physicians should abstain from framing hypotheses and theories about imperceptible things; whether randomized control trials are both necessary and sufficient to validate a therapy; whether medicine is science, technology, craft, or all three; whether complementary and alternative therapies deserve being included in medicine; whether placebos are purely imaginary or have biological effects; whether there are universal biomedical truths, or only social conventions; whether biomedical research is dominated by commercial interests and political power; and whether any of the best-known philosophers — Plato, Aristotle, Thomas Aquinas, Descartes, Spinoza, Locke, Hume, Kant, Hegel, Engels, Nietzsche, Mach, Russell, Husserl, Heidegger, Wittgenstein, Popper, and Foucault — have advanced medicine.

Moreover, an examination of medical praxis is likely to show that medics philosophize much of the time, even while claiming that philosophy bores them. Indeed, they practice logic when reasoning correctly; they tacitly embrace naïve realism when they take it for granted that patients, nurses, and pharmacies exist outside their minds; when they demand that hypotheses be checked against facts, they adopt scientific realism; they adopt a naturalistic worldview when they regard diseases as natural rather than as effects of divine curses or witchcraft; and when they treat patients even without being sure of collecting their fees, medics practice a humanistic moral philosophy. In short, medics — and paramedics and nurses and hospital administrators — philosophize just as spontaneously as they breathe.

The tacit occurrence of philosophy in medical practice does not prove that homespun philosophies suffice: let us remember Hippocrates' warning against what he called "postulates" (untested conjectures), in particular the fantasies of the pre-Socratic physicians and philosophers. The physician must always be on guard to filter the information barrages that the medical press and the medical visitor subject her to. In particular, she must be able to evaluate the claims to miracle cures and revolutionary medical theories. She must also be able to realize, or at least not to discard *a priori*, the medical potential of new biological, biochemical, and pharmacological findings.

Unless philosophy itself is toxic, it may help medics separate the grain from the chaff, as well as to organize the incoming information and spy the horizon. As well, philosophy may help craft overall views of medicine, like those proposed in earlier times by such intellectual leaders of the field as Philippe Pinel, Rudolf Virchow, Claude Bernard, Robert Koch, Paul Ehrlich, William Osler, Abraham Flexner, Peter Medawar, Lewis Thomas, and Thomas McKeown.

The aim of this book is to examine some of the conceptual issues raised by biomedical research and medical practice. For example, why are the traditional medicines mostly ineffective? Are diseases things (entities) or processes? Why do many medical diagnoses turn out to be wrong? What are the differences between molecular and classical pharmacology? Why are randomized clinical trials superior to non-randomized ones? Is evidence-based medical practice as novel as advertised? Is it correct to talk about probabilities in a field where there are neither objective randomness nor probabilistic theories? Are placebo effects purely imaginary? How might the current deadlock in the development of new drugs be overcome? Why has cancer medicine failed? Should medical assistance be rationed, and if so, how? Why do "complementary and alternative medicines" flourish in modern society? And what is to be done about the philosophical schools that deny reality and truth?

I am very grateful to Daniel Flichtentrei, MD (IntraMed), who encouraged, informed, and corrected me from the start. I am also indebted, for surgical interventions, to my colleagues Professor A. Claudio Cuello, MD; ScD, FRSC; Professor Ernesto Schiffrin, MD, PhD, FRSC; as well as to Nicolás Unsain, ScD. And I owe Enrique Mathov, MD and Bernard Dubrovsky, MD many years of enlightening exchanges.

My parents deserve special mention because both were health care workers, so that I grew up listening to medical cases, advances, and fads. My father, Dr. Augusto Bunge, had a passion for public health as a social good to be pursued by political means. My mother, Marie Müser, joined the German Red Cross at the age of 16 to train as a nurse and work in cholera-infested China. Both my parents taught me that the healing profession calls for mercy in addition to knowledge, dedication, and courage.

Finally, I owe valuable information to Professor Silvia Bunge, ScD; Professor Pierre Deleporte, ScD; José Luis Heraud, MD; Professor Michael Mackey, ScD, FRSC; Martin Mahner, ScD; Professor Carles Muntaner, MD, PhD; Adolfo Peña Salazar, MD; and Professor Amir Raz, PhD. Marta, my mathematician wife of 54 years, helped me in many ways, suggested the cover, and made plenty of suggestions — alas discarded in most cases. And I thank Joy Quek and Veronica Low for shepherding this book through the press with professionalism and patience.

Mario Bunge
Department of Philosophy
McGill University
Montreal, Canada

CONTENTS

INTRODUCTION

At first sight, medicine is alien to philosophy, since the former attempts to heal, or at least to alleviate pain, whereas philosophers analyze and systematize very general ideas, such as those of reality, knowledge, truth, and the good. In his *Ancient Medicine*, Hippocrates (430–420 B.C.) warned against philosophy. However, arguably, he only rejected the fantasies of the pre-Socratics, in particular the Pythagoreans, who had strongly influenced his precursors. Half a millennium later, his great disciple Galen opined that "the best doctor is also a philosopher."

As a matter of fact, medicine has always been saturated with philosophy, if only because medics cannot help using general ideas, such as those of reality and truth. Let us see how any contemporary physician philosophizes during a routine clinical examination. When the patient appears, the medic takes it for granted that she is a real being (*ontological realism*) who comes for help, something the doctor is willing to offer to the best of his ability and in accordance with the Hippocratic precept (*humanism*). To find out what ails her, the physician starts by asking her certain questions, whereby he tacitly admits that there is something he can get to know (*epistemological realism*), as well as something he can do to help her (*praxiological optimism*).

Thus, the contemporary physician does not believe that diseases are sent by a deity as punishment for sins, or by a sorcerer for sheer malice, and he regards medicine as an *ars vivendi*, not an *ars moriendi*. Moreover, he knows that death is the natural end of life, not God's punishment for Adam's original sin. In short, the modern medic adopts tacitly a secular worldview, and relies on biology rather than on theology. However, let us go back to the doctor's office.

The patient's replies to the doctor's initial questions may prompt additional questions, as well as a look at the patient's clinical history, which nowadays is just a click away — an ambivalent fact, because it results in the physician's looking more at the screen than at the person. But, far from believing everything the patient tells him, the doctor may doubt some of it (*methodological skepticism*). And he will try to translate into *signs* or *objective indicators* the *symptoms* that the patient feels — for instance, pains into lesions. Such translation of feelings into biomarkers betrays a *naturalist* view of disease, that is, the thesis according to which sickness symptoms are the subjective correlates of morbid bodily processes. To carry out such translations, the physician may have to use elements of the so-called medical technology, from the humble stethoscope to the sophisticated MRI (magnetic resonance imaging) apparatus. And he won't forget that there are neither isolated organs nor patients in a social vacuum (*systemism*).

As the medic absorbs the stream of data pertinent to the medical problem at hand, he keeps forming, evaluating, discarding, and replacing educated guesses (hypotheses about the nature of the disease and its possible causes). Zigzagging between data and hypotheses, he eventually hits on the conjectures that seem most plausible in the light of his knowledge and experience as well as of the data he has just collected.

These hypotheses are conditional propositions of the form "If the patient exhibits the sign or objective indicator S, then it is possible that she suffers disorder D." Except in the case of new diseases, the conjectures of this kind are not improvised, but occur in the standard medical literature. And they are neither arbitrary nor mere empirical rules, but are based on biomedical research, in particular controlled clinical trials. And this is a peculiarity of contemporary medical practice: that it is far more indebted to experiment than to dissection, to the laboratory working on living animals than to the post-mortem pathological study.

To find out which of his hypotheses is the truest, or at least the most plausible one, the medic reflects on what they imply, and he gets ready to check them. With luck, the answers to these questions will confirm one of his guesses. If not, he will order a few tests using some advanced diagnostic tools, such as blood analysis and X-rays. In principle, the diagnostic process continues until a clear (yet still fallible) answer is reached, and a prescription can be written.

In diagnosing as well as in prescribing, the contemporary medic applies tacitly the postulate that scientific research is the best means to get to know facts. This is the *scientism* postulate, first stated by Nicolas, Marquis de Condorcet on the eve of the 1789 French Revolution. In other words, our doctor tacitly rejects not only the magico-religious views, but also the intuitionism, apriorism, blind empiricism, and destructive skepticism inherent in postmodern constructivism-relativism, according to which there are no truths because there is no real world out there.

In short, our physician puts into practice the maxim *Learn before acting* (this is the slogan of scientific action theory, the rational alternative to pragmatism and Marxism). In complex cases, such as the ones handled by oncologists, immunologists, and psychiatrists, the treatment results will be so many additional data used to revise both the initial diagnosis and the corresponding treatment. The patient doubles then as an experimental guinea pig.

Such revisions are indicated not only when the diagnosis proves wrong, but also when the patient's immune system fails, as well as when a new drug has been used, whose efficiency has not yet been rigorously checked, or whose side effects are still poorly known. (Here is where the immoral practices of some pharmaceutical companies make themselves painfully felt.) So then, the responsible physician practices the rule that enjoins us to doubt and restart when something goes wrong.

This philosophical rule, *methodological skepticism*, should not be mistaken for radical or systematic skepticism, which rules out the possibility of ever attaining any certainty, even about the roundness of the Earth or the cause of pregnancies.

Finally, sometimes the physician faces moral problems. The toughest of all are the ones related to the beginning and the end of life, such a "Should one help bring to term a pregnancy with a fetus carrying a severe genetic defect?", "To save or not to save the very immature neonate, who has no chance of living a normal life?", "To prescribe or not a treatment that promises little and costs much?", and "To prolong or not the life of a terminal patient who can no longer enjoy life, let alone help others live?" In cases like these, the physician and his patient and next of kin will have to opt between some traditional moral philosophy and the humanist ethics condensed into the maxim *Enjoy life and help live*.

In sum, the good medic, in contrast to the shaman and the practitioner of an "alternative" medicine, practices, usually unwittingly, a whole philosophical system, containing

1) a materialist (though not physicalist) and systemic (though not holistic) ontology;
2) a rationalist, realist, skeptical, and scientificist epistemology; and
3) a science-based action theory and a humanist ethics.

This is the philosophy that the science-oriented medic practices, not necessarily the one he claims to profess. To check this diagnosis, imagine a physician who were to discard any of the three components listed above. For example, a spiritualist medic, such as a follower of homeopathy, whose founder claimed that a remedy is the more powerful the less matter it contains; or an anti-realist, like someone who holds that diseases are not biological disorders but social constructions, or that standard medicine is an invention of Big Pharma; or an anti-humanist, like the medics who experimented on inmates in prisons or camps, or on unsuspecting peasants, or those who oppose public health care. Who could trust any of these characters? The public should protect itself not only from medical delinquents and quacks, but also from antisocial sanitary politics and from sick philosophies. *Philosophia sana in ars medica sana.*

CHAPTER 1

TRADITIONAL MEDICINES

1.1 Primitive and Archaic Medicines

We do not know what primitive men thought or did about their health problems, beyond what little the study of their fossil remains and the accompanying artifacts may suggest. For example, we know that many primitives knew how to suture wounds and set broken bones, and that some of them practiced trephination. However, we do not know why they did the latter: whether to treat migraines or to release evil spirits.

By contrast, anthropologists have found out something about the ideas and practices of modern primitives. For example, the Amazonian Indians, who are among the most backward, use several plants to which they attribute healing or magic properties. Some tribes believe that they protect children from evil spirits by rubbing them with some plants. Others eat plants that, although poor in nutrition, are appreciated for their shape, color, or some other trait. This usage is enshrined in the doctrine of signatures, popular in Europe in the sixteenth and seventeenth centuries, according to which certain plants cure diseased organs because they resemble them in shape. And as recently as in the 1960s, Che Guevara, the physician turned revolutionary, was amazed to learn that his Congolese comrades believed that a certain magic potion had made them invulnerable to the colonialists' bullets.

A philosopher may think that the Amazonian tribesmen are dualists, in the sense that, while their practices are materialistic, their explanations are spiritualistic. Perhaps he will add that the Amazonians are half empiricists and half apriorists — the former because they learned their practices by trial and error, and the latter because other practices owe nothing to experience. For example, frequent bathing is an effective prophylactic habit,

1

whereas tribal mutilations, deformations, and scarifications are harmful, as is the insertion of thorns or bones in the skin.

We also know something about the medical beliefs and practices prevailing in the earlier civilizations, partly because some of them persist in ours. Despite their marked differences, all of them shared the belief that some or all diseases were caused by gods, evil spirits, or witchcraft (Trigger 2003: 620). Hence, sacrifices to supernatural entities were thought to help the application of natural remedies.

But in daily matters, it was always considered advisable to take practical measures, for the gods might be bribed and, in any event, they were busy with cosmic affairs. So, in practice, the sick person in the ancient world paid two fees: to his healer and to the god in charge of his particular disease. This was the ruling medical practice in all the early civilizations, whether in Eurasia, Africa, or America — a mixture of religious ceremony with more or less successful empirical practices (see, e.g., Mata Pinzón 2009; Sigerist 1961; Valdizán 2005; Varma 2011).

The Hippocratic, Ayurvedic, and traditional Chinese medicines, which had already peaked two millennia ago, stand out. They were the most important medical legacy of antiqutity because, though unscientific by modern standards, they broke with the magico-religious tradition; they were thoroughly secular and even materialist rather than spiritualist. Moreover, all three contained some nuggets of true knowledge and a few efficient practices, particularly concerning prophylaxis, diet, and lifestyle.

In the West, the Hippocratic school is the best known of all the traditional medical traditions. We owe to it the thesis that diseases are natural processes beyond the reach of the gods; that the disease of every kind has its own peculiar course; that most disorders heal without intervention; and that to keep well, as well as to recover health, we must observe certain simple hygienic rules, such as eating and drinking in moderation. We also owe the same school the attempt to find general laws and rules — an attitude common to all the sages of ancient Greece.

The ancient Egyptians had a lot of special mathematical and medical knowledge, but did not bequeath us a single general theorem or general medical rule. In particular, the famous Edwin Smith papyrus from 1,500 B.C. contains studies of 48 wounds in various parts of the body. The descriptions of the wounds and their treatments were detailed, objective, and rational. But they do not suggest any generalizations; they are strictly empirical, in contrast with the official ideology, which worshipped one god for every one of the 200 known diseases.

Empiricism is of course the sticking to experience and the corresponding rejection of magic and religious ideas. The same philosophy inspired also radical skepticism about theorizing, as exemplifed by the brilliant if destructive Sextus Empiricus. Radical skepticism was certainly reasonable at a time when almost all the extant theories were false or, as in the case of Aristotle's, they contained some religious ingredients.

Skepticism about scientific theories ceased to be reasonable and progressive when David Hume embraced it at the beginning of the eighteenth century, when classical mechanics was flourishing and the earliest biological and medical hypotheses emerged. Hume, an implacable critic of religion, also rejected Newtonian mechanics because it contained concepts, such as that of mass, that go beyond phenomena (appearances).

(This phenomenalism of Hume and his followers, from Immanuel Kant to Auguste Comte to Ernst Mach to Pierre Duhem to the logical positivists of around 1930, overlooked, opposed, or distorted all of the deep scientific theories, every one of which involves concepts referring to imperceptible entities and processes, from atoms and force fields to evolution and the innards of stars. Kant was well aware that phenomenalism is anthropocentric, but he was wrong in claiming that its adoption was "a Copernican revolution," for in fact it was a counter-revolution. Pierre Duhem realized this when he launched his attack on Galileo, whom he called "the Florentine mechanic," and proposed his own "physics of a believer.")

From the time of the consolidation of the scientific attitude, around 1800, empiricism was frankly regressive; it opposed all the bold new scientific theories, such as electrodynamics, atomism, and astrophysics, and it slowed down the renewal of medicine on the basis of chemistry, pharmacology, and biology. From then on, the philosophy that best favors the search for factual truth is what may be called *ratioempiricism*, which proposes a synthesis of reason with experience, as practiced in the experimental trial of medical hypotheses, such as those of the existence of oncogenes and of strong ties between the immune system and the rest of the body. However, let us go back to antiquity.

The transition from shamanism to Hippocratic medicine was slow and had an intermediate phase: the secular, rationalist, and materialist speculations of Thales, Empedocles, Anaxagoras, Democritus, Epicurus, and other pre-Socratics. These great thinkers speculated boldly, but they also argued and rejected the recourse to the magico–religious. Of course, the "elements" they imagined (water, air, soil, and fire) turned out to be complex, not elementary, and we now know that atoms do not move incessantly in a straight line. But we grant that the enormous variety of things around us comes from combinations of atoms of only 100 species, and that these constituents are material, not spiritual, as a consequence of which they are studied by physics and chemistry, not theology.

We all admire the great achievements of the Hippocratic school, but we must discard nearly all their explanations for, although they were rational and materialist, they were also speculative. In fact, the nucleus of the Hippocratic conception of disease is the hypothesis of the equilibrium of the four humors: blood, phlegm, yellow bile, and black bile. (The black bile, or *melaina chole*, has not been identified. It has been conjectured that it was an invention designed to satisfy the school's love of the number 4, which would also be the number of "elements.") Sickness would come from an imbalance of humors, which the medic has to correct. For example, if he suspects that there is an accumulation of blood in the feet, he will bleed them. (It would take two millennia to discover that blood circulates.)

Since not all humors are concentrated, neither are their disequilibria. This is why the humoral pathology is holistic. Therefore, so are the corresponding therapy and prophylaxis: the Hippocratic medic treated his patient as a whole. He prescribed global treatments: hygiene, diet, and lifestyle. This may have been the most lasting contribution of archaic Greek medicine: recommending good preventive habits.

Their holism did not prevent Hippocratic doctors from speculating about the functions of the few organs they distinguished. For example, Hippocrates adopted the hypothesis of the Sicilian medic Alcmaeon, that the brain is the organ of the mind, whereas the ancient Egyptians believed that the function of the brain is to secrete mucus, and Aristotle believed that its role was to cool down the blood, and the ancient Chinese held that the spleen is the organ of the mind.

Alcmaeon and Hippocrates were then the forerunners of biological psychology and psychiatry, the alternative to their magico-spiritualist, idealist, and dualist counterparts. They also inspired the popular classing of personalities (or temperaments or constitutional types) into phlegmatic, sanguine, and bilious.

With hindsight, it is easy to ridicule the humoral pathology. But it was the first to try and explain symptoms by proposing a concrete mechanism that involved only material entities, the four humors, three of which were familiar. Besides, this medical hypothesis, unlike the others, was not isolated but was part of a whole worldview that included another three quartets: Empedocles' four elements, the states warm–cold–dry–humid, and the four seasons. Those four constituents reinforced one another, which helps explain the popularity of Hippocratic medicine during two mllennia. (See Figure 1.1.)

The Ayurvedic and traditional Chinese medicines too were centered in equilibrium ideas. Three millennia ago, the Vedas postulated that every disease consists in an imbalance among three bodily systems — *vayu*, *pitta*, and *kapha* — which they did not bother to describe. Note their preference for the number 3, whereas the Greeks favored 4, the Mesopotamians 7, and the Chinese 2 and 5.

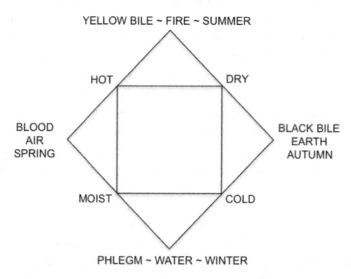

Fig. 1.1. The humoral pathology was part of a four-part cosmology (redrawn from Sigerist 1961, p. 323).

In all these cases, the medical theory fit the ruling worldview. But in the case of the Ayurvedics, this adjustment was only partial, as it ignored the tens of thousands of Hindu gods. And the corresponding therapy worked only with material means, such as salves and herbal teas, while the sacred scripture held that the universe is spiritual, whereas everything material is illusory. Nor is such duality rare or surprising: life must go on while paying the gods their due.

The followers of traditional Chinese medicine — just like the Ayurvedics and the Hippocratics — sought harmony. In their case, the desirable balance was that between the Yin and the Yang — an idea that agreed with Confucius' political principle of seeking social harmony. Those alleged basic properties were named but not described with any precision, and consequently they lent themselves to arbitrary interpretation. The same holds for the Qi (or *chi*), usually translated as "life force or energy," and is assumed to flow along the "meridians" or canals. These alleged anatomical entities are carefully drawn in the anatomic Chinese atlases produced for the past two millennia, but no modern anatomist has found them, and no physiologist has ever detected the Qi said to flow along them.

Suppose we are seen by a traditional Chinese doctor. What will he do to find out what ails us? He will examine our body, in particular the tongue and hands, in search of visible signs. He will put special attention to the shape and color of the tongue. If it is pale and swollen, and with a thick white coating, the diagnosis will be "Yang deficiency"; a red and cracked tongue will indicate "Yin deficiency"; and a pale and deformed tongue with teeth marks will be clear evidence that the patient is lacking in Qi. In turn, Yang deficiency indicates feeling cold and back pain; Yin deficiency indicates hot flashes and insomnia; and Qi deficiency points to fatigue and worry. Nothing seems to point to any of the most common infections or chronic diseases; it's all instant diagnosis of conditions one can live with.

Don't ask the traditional Chinese doctor what Yang, Yi, or Qi are, nor why Qi flows only along the "meridians"; nor what may obstruct the Qi flow, nor about the mechanism whereby a needle inserted in the right place will restore it. What matters is that the healer is sure that the said excesses or deficiencies occur and will be easily corrected by sticking needles at places invented two millennia ago, or by sipping infusions of certain herbs of unknown composition. He won't offer evidence of any sort, nor could he, given that he does not know what Yang, Yin, or Qi are, nor how they could be experimentally wiggled and measured. The traditional Chinese medic does not expect his patients to ask such questions, any more than a Christian priest expects his parishioners to ask him for evidence for resurrection. Both rely on the gullibility of their clients, who have been educated to believe without evidence and without explanation. There is no discovery in all that because there is no research — hence no research fraud. But at least traditional Chinese medicine is naturalistic rather than either shamanist or religious.

Chinese traditional medicine handles the human being as if he were an inscrutable *black box* with buttons and color lamps, and it treats its practitioner as a robot whose task it is to press buttons as indicated by a tradition-given code that pairs off colors with buttons. (This code is part of the *Yellow Emperor's Inner Laws*, the canon of the lore, composed between four and two centuries B.C.) Neither medic nor patient knows the nature of the sickness or the treatment. By contrast, scientific medicine and its practitioners look like *translucent* (or semitransparent) *boxes*: in principle everything can be examined, analyzed, tried out, and discussed. And no medical treatise is expected to be unalterable. Moreover, every day there is a medical novelty announced in the specialized journals, and consequently a significant part of the knowledge of today's medical graduate is expected to become obsolete in just five years from now.

In any event, since the traditional Chinese medic conceived of disease as an imbalance between the Yin and the Yang, his task consisted in guessing the said imbalances from symptoms, and in restoring the former — a task he attempted to carry out by performing acupuncture and prescribing massage, and diets including medicinal teas — of which there were more than 10,000 kinds. In this regard, in resorting exclusively to material means, the traditional Chinese medic was far superior to the shaman or priest. But in both cases what really worked, when it did, was presumably a placebo. Only experiment could say what, if anything, really worked. But experiment was invented two millennia after Chinese medicine was invented, and its contemporary practitioners do not experiment. (See Chapter 7.)

1.2 Achievements and Failures of Traditional Medicine

The above-mentioned hypotheses on balance or harmony are so imprecise, that they are untestable, hence unscientific. However, some of them can be refined and become the subject of experimental test. In particular, the modern version of the idea of bodily balance is the physiological concept of *homeostasis*, the constancy of the *milieu intérieur* that Claude Bernard conceived two millennia later, and Walter Cannon refined a century after Bernard.

One century after Bernard, it was found that the said balance results from negative feedback mechanisms. For example, the skin temperature is regulated by the hypothalamus, and the heart rhythm by the medulla oblongata. The search for bodily mechanisms is beyond traditional medicine, which at most delivered correct but superficial descriptions of overall processes, such as digestion.

Traditional medicine claimed to describe and explain all the known diseases (only modern medicine admits limitations). But it was unable to accomplish this task for lack of the biological knowledge required to correctly explain either the origin or the course of any disease. In sum, ancient medicine was nearly impotent because it was prescientific.

One might say that, contrary to Hippocrates' expectant and prudent attitude, the contemporary internal physician seeks to maintain or restore the normal values of the parameters that characterize the internal milieu of the healthy organism, such as temperature, blood pressure, acidity, and sugar and cortisol levels — all of them measurable and alterable by various means. (Incidentally, homeostasis, or "the wisdom of the body," as Cannon famously called it, goes only so far: sometimes the immune system "goes haywire," as is the case with the autoimmune disorders, from diabetes to AIDS.)

Besides, the ancient conjectures about bodily equilibrium, though imprecise and speculative, are materialistic, so that their advent was an enormous advance over the previous spiritualist fantasies (Varma 2011). This progress was not only conceptual but also practical because, if a disease is a natural fact, it may be treated by natural means — heat or cold, bath or compress, enema or herb tea, massage or knife, and so on — instead of either standing idly by waiting for the shaman's incantation, the sacrifice of a rooster to Aesculapius, or a visit to the health sanctuaries of Epidaurus or Lourdes to work.

In sum, the traditional Greek, Indian, and Chinese medicines were naturalistic. Hippocrates said so clearly: he held that nature cures as much as it sickens, whence the medic's task is to help nature along. The more-or-less explicit adoption of a materalist philosophy placed the earliest medicines proper at the margin of the ruling philosophy, which grew, albeit very slowly, in the shadow of the Christian and Islamic religions. This philosophical marginality allowed Western medicine to advance without paying much heed to the dominant religion or philosophy. Another factor that contributed to the independence of Western medicine with respect to the dominant ideology was its low social standing: medical practice was taken to be a mere craft and therefore no challenge to theology.

Finally, the Hippocratic postulate of the *vis medicatrix naturae* (healing power of nature) "was one of the greatest discoveries medicine could make" (Sigerist 1961: 326). First, because most diseases cure spontaneously thanks to the leukocytes synthesized by the bone marrow, the antibodies synthesized by the immune system, and other self-repairing mechanisms such as autophagy, or the digestion of damaged or redundant cells. For example, most inflammations and muscular pains disappear during the night; usually common colds do not last longer than a week; and brain concussions persist for only a few minutes to a few months. Second, that was a great discovery because in antiquity, when so little was known about the human body, drastic interventions could do more harm than good.

However, medics did not always observe Hippocrates' prudence. During two millennia, they routinely prescribed frequent bleedings, laxatives, diuretics, and emetics, along with drugs that turned out to be dangerous toxics. In the West, bleeding was applied enthusiastically between Galen's time and 1850, without any experimental evidence, to treat almost all diseases.

Until a century ago, the medicine chest of any Western middle-class family contained toxics like calomel (a mercury compound), taken regularly as a laxative; laudanum, an opiate used as analgesic; and belladonna, a powerful psychotropic that, in addition to alleviating pains, dilated the pupils of flirtatious ladies. Even nowadays, there is no shortage of physicians who prescribe piles of medicaments without first making sure that they do not interact among themselves, or whether a change in lifesyle, such as eating less and walking more, might suffice. In short, we are going through a hypermedication epidemic (Agrest 2011) — at least in the advanced nations. Much the same holds for surgery: much of it, especially in the USA, is unnecessary, as shown by statistical data (Groopman & Hartzband 2011). Surgery is much less frequent in the nations where medics are paid by the state.

The abuses of "official" medicine have provoked a resurgence of medical quackery, in particular homeopathy, acupuncture, and naturopathy. Such return to the past is just as irrational as giving up on democracy in view that it is limited, slow, and subject to corruption. The successful treatment of any disease is not less science but more of it combined with a moral conscience. For example, the recent success in curing AIDS patients is the result of high-level biomedical research. We shall come back to this subject in Section 1.3.

Finally, let us ask how effective the three main ancient medicines have been. This question has more than an antiquarian interest because all three are still being practiced nearly everywhere to the detriment of people, the flora, and the fauna. The current consensus seems to be as follows:

1) the medics of the Hippocratic and Ayurvedic schools proffered some good prophylactic advice, particularly concerning diet and personal hygiene;
2) some Hindu medics invented a few surgical procedures, particularly in plastic surgery, but of course they used neither asepsis nor anesthesia;
3) recent randomized controlled trials (e.g., Cherkin et al. 2009) have shown that acupuncture, the center of traditional Chinese medical medicine, is useless except as an analgesic placebo;
4) the Ayurvedic pharmacopeia is fantastic, since it contains about 7,000 medications to treat the 100 or so known medical signs, such as fever, diarrhea, and anemia;
5) only a few of the 11,000 Chinese medicinal herbs have been subjected to controlled clinical trials; for example, the *Cochrane Summaries* for July 8, 2009, inform that 51 studies on the anticarcinogenic action of green tea, involving 1.6 million subjects, were inconclusive; and it is known for sure that only a handful of Chinese medical herbs, among them the antimalarial artemisin, are effective;

6) contemporary scientific medicine makes no use of any of the three main traditional medicines beyond a few prophylactic and dietetic rules, and of the maxim *Do no harm*; and

7) the traditional medicines failed to distinguish symptom from sign or objective indicator; they measured no variables except for the amount of blood extracted; and they did not perform any clinical trials and kept no statistics, except for mortality during epidemics, and that only from the mid-seventeenth century on.

Before taking the next step, let us recall the crucial contribution of philosophy to the transition from traditional to modern medicine. The shift from myth to science, which attained maturity only at around 1800, was not sudden but extremely slow, and it was marked by an important middle phase: the rational and materialist speculation of the likes of Thales, Anaxagoras, Empedocles, Democritus, Epicurus, and other great pre-Socratic thinkers. These philosopher-scientists speculated, but they also offered reasons and rejected magic and religion. Besides, they sketched a naturalist (or materialist) worldview that favored medicine because it assumed that all diseases, even the mental ones, are natural processes, and because it did not revile the body.

As we noted earlier, we now know that the "elements" that Empedocles imagined are not simple, but we agree that they are material rather than spiritual. We also know that nature "obeys" laws, and that the belief in lawfulness helped get rid of belief in witchcraft, divine arbitrariness, and destiny. This new attitude helped replacing consulting oracles and accumulating isolated data with the search for regularities — laws of nature and man-made behavior patterns, in particular health care practices.

This combination of rationality with materialism and with the realistic principle of the autonomous existence, lawfulness, and intelligibility of the universe was unique and it was modern *avant la lettre*. This may also have been the main contribution of pre-Socratic philosophy. It was indeed a new way of looking at things and exploring them, that overcame confusions, obscurities, fantasies, and irrational fears. What a contrast to the obscurantism and pessimism of the self-styled postmoderns, in particular the radical skeptics and the constructivist-relativists! These philosophers inhibit the search for truth because they deny that it is possible and

Table 1.1. The main traits of the process that transformed the mythical into the scientific intellectual culture. Think of the following sequences: Hesiod–Thales–Galileo, and Mythico-religious–Hippocratic–Scientific medicine.

Aspect	Phase
Logical	Confusion → Rational argument → Exact concepts.
Ontological	Mythology → Speculative materialism → Scientific ontology.
Epistemological	Dogma → Plausible conjecture → Confirmed hypothesis.

desirable; they suspect that scientific research is a political conspiracy, and attempt to pass off obscurity for profundity. Some of them also believe that the world is "a text or like a text" (see, e.g., Balibar & Rajchman 2011). However, let us go back to the fresh and productive speculations of the pre-Socratics.

The phase of philosophical speculation intermediate between magical and scientific thinking covered three aspects: logical (rationality), onto-logical (naturalism), and epistemological (realism). (See Table 1.1.)

Contrary to received wisdom, the Indian thinkers of the same period thought very similar ideas (Tola & Dragonetti 2008). And it is possible that they contributed to the traditional Indian medicine being just as secular and naturalistic as their Greco-Roman counterparts. On the other hand, the Indian philosophers did not help the birth of science, perhaps because the Vedas, the Indian sacred scriptures, had a ready-made answer to everything. The ancient Greeks, by contrast, were not smothered by a detailed religious worldview and were not watched by a priestly caste, so they were free to ask questions of all kinds and to answer them with little censorship. This is how, between the sixth and the fifth centuries B.C., the pre-Socratic philosophers emerged, who generated not only medicine but also science, the branch of culture that flourished only in Greece. Yes, the Greek Miracle did happen, but of course it was wholly man-made, it did not last long, and research — the mark of science — did not touch medicine until the Scientific Revoluton of around 1600, to be examined in the next chapter. Let us now take a look at some fossils of the primitive and archaic healing arts.

1.3 Contemporary Medical Quackery

What became of the primitive and archaic medicicines? They are still with us under the name of *complementary and alternative medicines*, or CAMs for short. This is a broad panoply of therapies lacking in both scientific basis (knowledge of mechanism) and evidence (randomized controlled trials). The vast majority of the practitioners of these "alternative" medicines — or rather alternatives to medicine — are individuals without a medical background, or MDs who conceal their university diplomas so as not to shoo away people who distrust science.

Most inhabitants of the so-called developing nations seek the help of medical quacks. In the USA, nearly half the population resorts to "unconventional" medicines, in particular chiropractic, homeopathy, acupuncture, and herbalism — despite the warnings of *Consumer Report,* which people consult and listen to before buying really important things, such as cars and domestic appliances.

Some CAM therapies, in particular the herbalist, Ayurvedic, and traditional Chinese ones, are thousands of years old. Others, like homeopathy, chiropractic, iridology, and osteopathy, are far more recent. Let us briefly examine three of the most popular CAMs: holism, homeopathy, and naturopathy.

Holism is one of the New Age slogans, for it suggests the opposite of analysis and reason, which in turn are targets of the enemies of modernity. Holistic medicine, usually advertised as novel, is nothing of the sort. Indeed, treating the patient as a whole is a characteristic of the primitive and ancient internal medicines: they *had* to treat patients as black boxes because they knew neither anatomy, nor physiology, nor biochemistry. By contrast, scientific medicine treats patients like translucent boxes, that is, systems that can be dismantled, at least conceptually, with the help of modern biology: it is *systemic.*

The conceptual or empirical analysis of a concrete system, from atom to body to society, consists in identifying its composition, environment, structure, and mechanism. These components may be schematically defined as follows:

Composition = Set of constituents on a given level (molecular, cellular, etc.)

Environment = Immediate surrounding (family, workplace, etc.)

Structure = Set of bonds among the components (ligaments, hormonal signals, etc.)

Mechanism = Process(es) that maintain(s) the system as such (cell division, metabolism, circulation of the blood, etc.)

This analysis evokes six groups of ontological (metaphysical) doctrines, some of which have an ancient pedigree:

Environmentalism The environment is omnipotent. Examples: behaviorism, and the hypotheses that all diseases are caused by either "miasmas" or social conditions.

Structuralism A whole is a network — the set of connections among its parts. Examples: connectionist psychology, and the sociological thesis that only communication networks matter — as if there could be graphs without nodes.

Processualism A concrete thing is a bunch of processes. Example: Alfred North Whitehead's metaphysics.

Holism The whole precedes and dominates its parts. Examples: Aristotle's metaphysics and traditional Asian medicines.

Individualism A whole is the set of its parts. Examples: ancient atomism and the thesis that health depends exclusively on the individual's habits — whence sanitary policies are useless and therefore wasteful.

Systemism The universe is the system of all systems. Examples: d'Holbach (1770), Bertalanffy (1950), and Bunge (1979).

The first five doctrines are logically incorrect. Holism and individualism are mistaken because the concepts of whole and part define one another: one cannot exist without the other. Environmentalism is false because every concrete thing is active: it is certainly influenced by its environment but not wholly generated by it. Structuralism is false because, by definition, there is no network without nodes (individuals). Lastly, processualism too is wrong because every process (e.g., growth) is a sequence of states of some concrete thing: neither processes without things nor immutable things.

In conclusion, only systemism remains of all the six structural ontologies listed above. (In addition, there are three possible substance ontologies: materialism, spiritualism, and dualism.) This ontology, initially proposed in the mid-Enlightenment by Paul-Henri Thiry, Baron d'Holbach, postulates that every really (materially) existing thing is a system or a component of some system. Arguably, systemism is the ontology that fits the modern sciences, from quantum physics and biology to psychology and historiography (Bunge 2012a). And, because it entails emergentism, systemism overcomes reductionism in its various forms, in particular mechanism, biologism, and sociologism.

Scientific medicine too is systemic because it is based on anatomy and physiology, which show that the parts of the body, though distinct, are interconnected. For example, the brain ceases to feel, think, and decide normally when not well irrigated; and reading a word, a process that occurs in the parietal cortex, may evoke a visual image in the back of the brain. And hormones of various kinds, which carry chemical "messages," reach every part of the body.

But of course, scientific medicine is analytic as well as systemic, in that it distinguishes distinct organs, every one of which has specific functions, that is, processes that occur only in them. Morever, *systemicity implies analyticity*, for understanding a system involves analyzing it. Systemicity also includes the valid component of holism, namely the thesis that "a whole is more than the set of its parts," in that a system possesses global properties that its parts lack.

These global or systemic properties are usually called *emergent* (see Bunge 2003a). Examples: solid state and the property of being alive. All the diseases are emergent processes because they occur only in initially healthy organisms, even though some of them, such as cancer and Down syndrome, have molecular roots, whereas others, notaby stress, have social causes.

Caution: the preceding definition of *emergence* differs from that given by the standard dictionaries, according to which emergent is whatever defies analysis. Following this definition, "emergence" would be an epistemological category (or belonging to knowledge), not an ontological one (belonging to the world). For example, the radical reductionists, from Epicurus onward, held that there is no death because the elementary constituents of an organism are conserved. And Richard Dawkins found the very existence of organisms paradoxical, since only genes would matter. Actually, only a biology without *bios* would be paradoxical.

Evidently, the structure of a system — that is, the set of connections among its parts — is just as important as the latter. For instance, a cell dies — it becomes a collection of molecules when its membrane disintegrates and stops synthesizing proteins and metabolizing. The property of being alive is emergent, as are the properties of thinking and socializing. And the emergent properties are peculiar to systems, in contradistinction to collections or sets.

To better understand the relations and differences between the analytic and the systemic, it helps comparing a modern anatomical atlas with a medieval one. In the latter, the organs were disconnected from one another, whereas in a modern atlas they are shown interconnected, some directly and others through the brain, which acts as the central control system. Besides, modern medics examine and treat their patients at all levels, from the molecular to the social. For example, a routine blood analysis includes the identification of certain proteins, and a clinical consultation may involve finding out facts about family, work, and even neighborhood conditions. And just moving to a better neighborhood can have a strong and lasting effect on subjective well-being (Sampson 2012). Moral: look for both *bottom-up* and *top-down* streams.

In sum, modern medicine is systemic and thus analytic as well, whereas traditional medicine was holistic. When claiming to treat the patient as a whole, the traditional healer missed the peculiarities of the parts. This feature explains the ineffectiveness of the holistic therapies, since the membranes of all cells contain *receptors*, all of which are specific, that is, systems that are stimulated or inhibited (blocked) only by molecules of certain types. For example, sildenafil, the active drug of Viagra, acts only on the penis, whereas the aphrodisiacs act only on receptors in brain cells of both sexes. The opiate receptors are widely distributed in the nervous system. By contrast, the insulin receptors are far more commonly distributed in the body; they are found in muscle and adipose tissues because of the affinity of insulin for sugar, the body's energizer.

The drugs that act on receptors of more than one type are called "dirty." A typical "dirty" drug is the antidepressant chlorpromazine, the first antipsychotic to be synthesized. Since "dirty" drugs affect not only their intended targets but also unintended receptors, they have side effects, in some cases adverse, but in others beneficial. For example, chlorpromazine acts also as a tranquilizer and as an anti-addictive, and codeine relieves pain but also induces euphoria.

Almost all known receptors are proteins, and these are molecules at least 100 times bigger than the classical drugs. (The so-called *biologics*, synthesized by the immune system or extracted from living things, are far bigger molecules.) The shape and electric charge of receptors fit only a few out of the millions of known molecules: this is why they are highly selective, that is, have no affinity with the rest.

This selectivity is a natural selection mechanism. An organism incapable of distinguishing beneficial from harmful molecules would be unviable. Incidentally, the existence of selective receptors refutes Nietzsche's opinion that a morality "beyond good and evil" favors life. Before the emergence of organisms, around 3,500 million years ago, there was neither good nor evil in the universe — which is why physics and chemistry do not use the concept of natural value.

Let us go back to the mechanism of action of medicaments, for it is highly relevant to the distinction between CAMs and medicine proper. The incident molecule, such as that of a drug, is effective only if it fits the receptor enzyme: this is the *lock-and-key* mechanism. This explains why the vast majority of modern medicaments are *specific*, that is, they act only on some parts (e.g., tissues or organs) of the body or on certain pathogens. For example, adrenaline stimulates the heart because the membrane of the heart cells contains adrenaline receptors, which do not occur in other organs.

The specificity of such receptors also explains the mechanism of action of what Paul Ehrlich, their discoverer, called "magic bullets." These drugs only kill certain pathogenic organisms. For example, Salvarsan, invented in 1910 by the same scientist, was the earliest effective drug against syphilis. The receptors, of which more than 2,000 species are known, constitute the clue to scientific pharmacology, in contradistinction to the traditional and modern "alternative" medicines, all of which ignore the very existence of receptors.

Admittedly, the preceding is an oversimplification, since many molecules are effective only when in the company of others. In other words, in many cases it is not enough to activate (stimulate or inhibit) a given receptor, but it is necessary to activate simultaneously another two or more receptors — which should not be surprising in a systemic perspective. Still, in all cases, what counts is not the entire organism but only a minute part of it. Let this be a warning against holism, which claims to treat the whole body while ignoring every part of it.

Let us turn to other CAMs, starting with the most absurd of them all. *Homeopathy* is not holistic, except in that it ignores the whole of science, for it admits the need to use specific medicaments. But the homeopathic specifics are imaginary, since homeopaths neither conduct nor use pharmacological studies showing the effectiveness of their nostrums at the molecular level. Nor do they carry out clinical trials to check whether their patients do better than those of the "allopaths." Indeed, they indulge all the time in the *post hoc, ergo propter hoc* ("after that, hence because of that") fallacy. The ancients ridiculed this fallacy by referring to the rooster who believed that he caused the Sun to rise when he crowed.

Moreover, homeopaths do not do any research; they only apply the "laws" that Samuel Hanemann stated two centuries ago, and they compile anecdotes of alleged cures — but, of course, they do not keep track of their failures. Furthermore, homeopaths do not use any of the diagnostic tools of "allopathic" (modern) medicine, such as the microscope, X-rays, and biochemical, bacteriological, and parasitological analyses. Nor do they check the effectiveness of their remedies, which nowadays are manufactured by big companies that do not invest in research. All their alleged medicaments are high dilutions of "active principles," mostly of vegetal origin. These dilutions are so high, that what the patient buys is nearly pure water or, in the case of pills, nearly pure excipient.

In fact, a homeopathic remedy is prepared by successive dilutions of a natural product — vegetal, animal, or mineral. At every step, a hundredth part of the remains of the previous step are extracted and poured in a flask containing 99 drops of alcohol. Thus every time, one-hundredth of the previous quantity is obtained. For example, in dilution No. 5, only $(1/100)^5 = 10^{-10}$ of the initial amount remains; and after 30 dilutions, the number recommended by the father of homeopathy $(1/100)^{30} = 10^{-60}$ remains — which is less than one molecule per galaxy (see Sanz 2010). Whereas existentialists believe that all is nothing, homeopaths believe that nothingness is everything.

Of course, one often hears of healing due to homeopathic treatments. But, since homeopaths do not conduct any controlled experiments, one must suspect that the improvement, if real, was the work of their immune system — or of the ubiquitous and ever serviceable Doctor Placebo, as Shang *et al.* (2005) proved. And, even if the (unknown) percentage of positive cases were appreciable, one should not discard the (unknown) number of deaths caused by the non-intervention of standard medicine. For instance, the unchecked proliferation of cancer cells is caused by the inhibition of apoptosis (programmed cellular death), whose molecular root cannot be affected by a few drops of colored water. In the case of a homeopathic treatment, due to the negligible amounts of supposedly active principle, there is no possible biological mechanism mediating between input and output: there is only illusion. In short, homeopathy is a black box with water, money, and illusion coming in, and money and self-deception as outputs.

Our second example of a CAM will be *naturopathy*. This is a component of *naturism*, which in turn is the philosophical doctrine that everything evil comes from deviating from nature. Naturism should not be mistaken for *naturalism*, the ontology that rejects the supernatural and holds the identity of the universe with nature, as well as the reduction of everything human to animality (see, e.g., Krikorian 1944; Shook & Kurtz 2009; Mahner 2012). Whereas naturalism is a worldview, naturism is basically a value judgment: "The natural is better than the artificial."

Naturism, a part of the Stoic philosophy that flourished in ancient Greece and Rome, was revived by Rousseau in the eighteenth century, and was continued in the next by the German Romantics, in particular Goethe, whose lemma was "Back to nature!" In the twentieth century, naturism was involved in three very different social movements: anarchism, the youth movement (eventually hijacked by the Nazis), and radical (or "deep") ecologism.

The popularity of naturism in Germany did not affect the eclosion of pharmacology in the same country. But, when joined with Nietzsche's vitalism, naturism acquired political partners one century after Romanticism: anarchism in the Latin countries, and Nazism in the Germanic realm. It also changed the lifestyles of millions of youths, who adopted vegetarianism, camping, nudism, a sexual morality without duties, and anti-intellectualism. (Note the paradoxical similarities with the "hippie" movement in the 1960s.)

The radical (or "deep") ecologism of the late twentieth century inverted the biblical myth that nature is God's gift to man; it held that, quite on the contrary, humankind should sacrifice itself for nature. In particular, the polluting industries, such as mining and the chemical industries, should be eliminated. This campaign has had a positive result: it has stimulated the development of "green chemistry," which seeks to replace the same products using less polluting reactants than the standard or "brown" chemistry, which is perfectly possible in many cases. It also flagged the mining industries that are causing irreversible environmental disasters, in contaminating the soil and water sources. In sum, there is a rational and feasible alternative to both radical ecologism and the untrammeled exploitation of nature taught by the Bible. However, it is time to get back to CAMs.

The case of naturopathy is epistemologically similar but ontologically dissimilar to that of homeopathy: both involve the ignorance of the scientific method, but the former handles causes, and consequently obtains some effects. Indeed, unlike the proverbially minute and therefore innocuous homeopathic doses, the natural remedies in reasonable doses are incorporated into the metabolism and thus alter it to some extent. Even a cup of mint tea has some effect — roughly that of a glass of water in addition to a placebo effect. Besides, when boiling water, one kills the myriad bacteria contained in the water extracted from wells or ponds.

Roughly half of the 100 most-used pharmaceutical drugs have a vegetal origin. It is also true that the drinks made from a few herbs have some beneficial effects at short range. But some popular natural products have adverse effects, some directly and others because they interact with pharmaceutical drugs (De Smet 2002). For example, licorice, ginseng, and valerian are toxic, and St. John's wort, which used to be recommended for mild depression, interferes with oral contraceptives and other drugs. In any case, the few rigorous clinical trials of natural products have been conducted by scientists, not by naturopaths. None of the thousands of trials published in journals of traditional Chinese medicine have been rigorous (Tang et al. 1999).

Every time a medic considers prescribing a natural product, she should ask two questions: which, if any, are the adverse effects of that product, and what is the suitable dose? (The biomedical researcher will add a third question: which is its mechanism of action?) But the sale of such products is not regulated because it is usually believed that, being natural, they must be as harmless as kitchen vegetables. Unlike the herbalist, the manufacturer of synthetic remedies has the legal obligation of responding to those two questions on the strength of laboratory assays and clinical trials.

Now, the trial of natural remedies is a very hard task because every herb, root, seed, bark, or mushroom contains molecules of dozens of different kinds. Hence, unless they are identified and tried one by one, it is impossible to find out which is the "active principle" and which, if any, are the harmful molecules.

(Incidentally, molecules cannot cause anything since, by definition, causes and effects are events, not things. The cause in question, when it exists, is the incorporation of the molecule as a reagent in a metabolic process or some more basic process, such as the stimulus or inhibition of some protein. Again, the National Rifle Association is right in holding that guns do not kill. But it is egregiously wrong in claiming that the availability of guns does not increase the likelihood of using them to kill — which is their only possible use.)

Because the composition of a natural product is never known in detail, one cannot know all the biochemical mechanisms that it triggers, accelerates, or slows down when ingested. This ignorance justifies the naturopaths' proceeding by trial and error rather than using the scientific method, which they reject anyway. By contrast, when the composition of a substance and the salient traits of the disease it is expected to interfere with are known, one may frame and test precise hypotheses about the possible outcomes of the action of the substance in question.

Still, in recent years, some heterodox therapies have been subjected to rigorous clinical trials. In particular, between 1999 and 2009, the National Institutes of Health have invested millions of taxpayers' dollars in checking the effectiveness of a variety of "alternative" therapies, from "healing at a distance" to Vedic and Chinese medicaments, magnetic fields, and many herbs and mushrooms, without any positive results (Mielczarek & Engler 2012). The methodological moral is obvious: trial and error is intellectually sloppy and socially wrong. But only hypotheses compatible with the bulk of scientific knowledge should be subjected to time-consuming and expensive clinical tests. Besides, such trials should be paid for by the companies that peddle natural products; this is demanded by the methodological principle that those who make a claim should bear the burden of its proof. At any rate, scientific breakthroughs occur within science, not against it.

The above does not involve rejecting out of hand all the natural products. We know that some of them are therapeutically effective, and that others contain molecules employed in the synthesis of drugs. But others, such as ephedra and aconite, have proved to be toxic. One-fifth of the most frequently prescribed Japanese medical herbs have been found to be toxic (Sakurai 2011).

It is also known that *all* therapies are effective to some extent, due to two factors. One of them is the *vis medicatrix naturae*, or spontaneous recovery, so highly valued by the Hippocratic school, and whose mechanisms are being investigated by immunology. The second factor that enhances the virtues of any treatment is the set of placebo effects. These are real even when the placebo objects, such as prayer and homeopathic water, do not act at the molecular level. (More on this in Chapter 7.)

In conclusion, the CAMs handle products of unknown nature (composition and structure), that they apply to persons who have not been properly studied, and with effects whose kind and intensity are not well known. They start from ignorance, act in ignorance, and come back to it. The circuit is: ? → ? → ?

The CAMs are just as groundless and ineffective as the traditional ones, with some important differences. First, whereas the latter contained some reasonable prophylactic and dietetic rules, the CAMs have contributed nothing true or useful to health care. Second, whereas the traditional medicines were artisanal and transmitted mainly through oral means, the modern CAMs are coupled to big pharmaceutical companies and are being intensely publicized. Third, medical superstition was justified at a time when there was no biomedical research, but nowadays the latter is highly developed, so that what used to be mere involuntary error is now large-scale swindle.

How to explain the popularity of the pseudosciences in such an important, well-cultivated, and regulated field as health care? Like any other social fact, this one has multiple causes. Here are some of them.

1) The CAMs constitute the medicine of those who ignore the scientific method, and these are the vast majority in any society.

2) Any pseudoscience can be learned in a few days, whereas learning any science or technology takes many years.

3) CAM is the medicine of the patients abandoned by "official" medicine, which has not yet been able to heal them; for example, Paul Feyerabend, of "Anything goes" fame, suffered intense back pain until he met a London witch who cured him; this experience was enough to sweep away all his science and all his philosophy of science.

4) Cultural relativism, which is often preached in the name of open-mindedness, denies the possibility of finding objective and universal truths, so that it holds that the differences between shamanism and scientific medicine are cultural or ideological. The influential Flexner Report (1910) devoted a long chapter to a severe condemnation of what it called "medical sects," among which it included homeopathy and osteopathy, and it criticized "tolerance" in matters of health care. One century later, some universities have forgotten that report and are now teaching those pseudosciences — the medical equivalent of decriminalizing crime.

5) Many people mistrust the pharmaceutical industry because it lives off suffering and because some Big Pharma firms have been guilty of inexcusable mistakes and crimes, such as bribing doctors so that they would prescribe drugs that failed to pass rigorous trials, such as Thalidomide, Vioxx, Avandia, Avastin, and other harmful drugs. (In 2009 Pfizer was fined US$2.3 billion, and in 2012 GlaxoSmithKline US$3 billion for such crimes.) But obviously blaming some companies should not involve rejecting pharmacology.

6) Counterculture and its academic counterpart, postmodernism — cultivated mainly in faculties of humanities — are consumed by a broad sector of people who feel disgusted by whatever smells of science.

7) Academic obscurantism, in particular the rejection of the intellectual ideals of the French Enlightenment (rationality, scientism, and progressivism). Such obscurantism, which until the 1960s was typical of political conservatism, is now shared by self-styled leftists who judge science from a political viewpoint instead of doing politics informed by social science.

8) The yellow press and publishers of all stripes, including some university presses, have spread plenty of texts that reject rationality and the

scientific method, such as the bestsellers *Ageless Body* and *Timeless Spirit*.

9) The UN's World Health Organization (WHO) acknowledges that "Evaluation of quality, safety and efficacy based on research is needed to improve approaches to assessment of traditional medicines," and yet it "urges national governments to respect, preserve and widely communicate traditional medical knowledge" (WHO 2011). And the National Institutes of Health invest US$128 million per year in CAMs. In short, medical quackery, that used to be a part of folklore, now comes also from above.

10) Political conservatism breeds scientific obscurantism, like that of former U.S. President George W. Bush when he opposed the medical use of stem cells and pushed for the replacement of evolutionary biology with the religious doctrine of "intelligent design." This provoked his successor, Barack Obama, to declare: "We have watched as scientific integrity has been undermined and scientific research politicized in an effort to advance predetermined ideological agendas" (White House 2010).

In conclusion, the pseudosciences are more popular than the sciences because gullibility is far more widespread than critical thinking, which is not acquired by compiling and memorizing data, but rethinking what had been learned. It is surely a duty of scientists, technologists, physicians, philosophers, and journalists to expose the frauds of CAMs, as Martin Gardner (1957), Robert Park (2000), R. Barker Bausell (2007), Ben Goldacre (2010), and a few others have done, as well as the *Skeptical Inquirer* magazine and the *Quackwatch.com* site. The CAMs are sects: they combine dogmatism (the refusal to face facts and debate rationally) with radicalism. And, of course, sectarianism is dangerous in all walks of life, particularly in politics and in health matters.

And it is the duty of public health oufits, such as the WHO, as well as of medical schools, to protect the public from medical quackery, starting by canceling the accreditation of universities that teach CAMs. This measure was taken in the USA on a national scale when the Carnegie Foundation published its report on medical education in the USA and Canada (Flexner 1910). But since then, the medical pseudosciences have recently reappeared around the world, even in prestigious universities, often in the name of openness. Evidently, tolerance is indicated within science, as well as in matters of taste or opinion. Morever, we should celebrate scientific and technological heterodoxy, for it is nothing but great originality. But we should be intolerant to medical charlatanry because it is bad for health and it degrades culture (Bunge 1996b).

Coda

The history of medicine may be divided into four periods: primitive, archaic, early modern, and contemporary. Primitive medicine, practiced by shamans who claimed to possess extraordinary faculties, and who often wielded great cultural and political power, mixed magico-religious superstitions with effective recipes to heal wounds and treat a few diseases. They gave analgesics, laxatives, and emetics; they bandaged, sutured, or cauterized wounds and set broken bones; and they sucked the poison injected by snakes and insects. But sometimes they also took and prescribed hallucinogens, or claimed to heal wounds by smearing them with excrements or by applying salves on the weapons that had caused them.

The archaic medicines that emerged in the early civilizations were far superior: they were wholly secular and gave some good advice, such as bed rest, keeping clean, and eating and drinking in moderation, but they also prescribed herbs and ointments that were innocuous in the best of cases. The traditional Chinese medics abused their needles, which were totally useless and sometimes propagated bacteria. And the Hindu medics prescribed thousands of vegetal derivatives without any proven therapeutic value.

The most rational of the ancient medics were those of the schools of Hippocrates and Galen, famous for their prudence and for giving some good prophylactic and dietetic advice, from bed rest to drinking only barley water. But neither these physicians nor the shamans could use anatomy or physiology, for these sciences were born in early modern times.

In the ancient Greco-Roman world, the birth and development of medicine proper were favored by the naturalist ontology of the pre-Socratic and Stoic philosophers, as well as by the rationalism and scientism of Aristotle and his disciples, mainly Theophrastus and Alexander of Aphrodisias. In ancient India, the rationalism and naturalism of the

Chárvaka, Sämkhya, and Jain schools played a similar constructive role, except that in that country, scientific research emerged only during the twentieth century. But at least traditional (Ayurvedic) Indian medicine, like the Hippocratic and Galenic schools, kept free from magic and religion.

Creative and secular intelligence became all but extinct with the rise of Christianity in the West, and with the Mongol conquest in India a millennium later. In both cases, scientific curiosity and rational debate about worldly matters ceased almost completely during these centuries, until they reappeared in the West with the Renaissance. (In Asia, modernity was involuntarily carried by European colonialism — along with some diseases.) Medicine and philosophy were, of course, important parts of those processes of development, decadence, and rebirth. In the next chapter, we shall review the radical changes in medicine since the Scientific Revolution that started around 1550. This deep cultural transformation wiped off the cobwebs of tradition, which from then on was seen as deserving to be studied but not worshipped.

CHAPTER 2

MODERN MEDICINE

2.1 From Myth to Science

The Hippocratic stance, of abstaining from intervening when one does not know what is going on in a patient, was exceptional and admirable at a time when tradition, dogmas, and oracles were far more appreciated than the reflections of the rare skeptical philosophers. The meticulous clinical stories of the Hippocratics, and later on of Galen's followers, were exemplary for their precision, concision, and clarity. They prepared the ground for the emergence of medical science, which started two millennia later along with anatomy and physiology and, much later, chemistry, bacteriology, and virology.

What characterizes modern medicine is scientific research, which combines precise observation with bold hypothesizing and demanding experiment. Yet, from 1990 on, there has been much talk, both pro and con, of *evidence-based* medicine, or EBM. The founders of this movement have characterized it thus: "Evidence based medicine is the conscientious, explicit, and judicious use of current best evidence in making decisions about the care of individual patients. The practice of evidence based medicine means integrating individual clinical expertise with the best available external clinical evidence from systematic research." (Sackett *et al.* 1996)

Undoubtedly, this demand for empirical rigor is an antidote to the dogmatism of yore, a challenge to the blind faith in experience and the "clinical eye," and even a defense against business irresponsibility. So much so, that a representative of Merck Sharp & Dohme, and another of Schering Plough, had the impudence to declare that the worst trait of EBM is "its limiting, blocking and controlling side" (Freddi & Román-Pumar 2011), which is like saying that the trouble with penal law is that it deters and punishes crime.

In this writer's opinion, the only objectionable traits of EBM are that it is not as novel as its champions claim it to be, and that it exaggerates the weight of evidence at the expense of that of hypothesis. In fact, the historians of medicine inform us that respect for empirical evidence was born two and a half millennia ago in the Hippocratic school, and that it came of age in Paris at the beginning of the nineteenth century, not in Hamilton, Canada, at the end of the twentieth century. Suffice it to recall the pioneering work of Xavier Bichat (histology), René Laënnec (stethoscope), Gaspard Bayle (tisiology), Philippe Pinel (biological psychiatry and humane psychiatric hospitals), and Pierre Louis (quantitative medicine). This is why, during the first half of the nineteenth century, Paris was the Mecca of medical students: because it was the world center of scientific medicine. In short, a quick look at the history of medicine (e.g., Kiple 1993; Porter 1996, 1997) suffices to learn that *all* the medicines proper, from Hippocrates' on and by contrast to shamanism, have *always* sought and used empirical data about sick people and their surroundings.

Despite the fact that EBM is more than two millennia old, the inventors of the name EBM insist on using it; they claim that the use of therapies that have not passed randomized clinical trials not only puts population at risk, but is also one of the causes of the ever higher cost of health care. For want of empirical data, we shall not examine this hypothesis about medical economics, but shall confine our attention to some of the philosophical problems posed by EBM.

For starters, note the difference between *evidence* and *datum*. Taken in themselves, data are neutral: they prove nothing. A datum becomes evidence when confronted with a hypothesis: in this case it either confirms or weakens the hypothesis to some extent. For example, a patient's body mass index is just a datum but, if excessive, it points to the risk of diabetes, a condition that can only be ascertained by looking for further data, such as sugar level in the blood.

In emphasizing the weight of tests, the champions of EBM involuntarily forget that the most important scientific findings are not gotten by piling up data, but by combining data with educated guesses and, more precisely, by designing observations and experiments in the light of plausible hypotheses about the possible mechanisms underlying the data.

Research guided by ideas is surely superior to mindless data gathering, just as agriculture is more effective than food collection.

What would Christopher Columbus have found if he had taken a zigzag course? It is likely that his supplies of food and drinking water would have been exhausted before finding land. And would Paul Ehrlich have founded modern pharmacology if he had analyzed or combined substances at random to see what happens, the way children like to do when given chemistry sets? Of course not. Ehrlich conjectured that every type of living tissue has affinity for drugs of a certain kind, because it has receptors that combine with them and not others. For example, muscle tissue has receptors for curare, and nervous tissue for opiates. No receptor hypothesis, no modern pharmacology — hence no contemporary therapy either.

What really changed radically from around 1800, and not 1990, are the *quality* and *use* of biomedical data. Let us see.

1) Whereas before the contemporary period only case studies (clinical histories) were used as data sources, in recent times findings of biomedical *research* (laboratory and clinical trials) are also used, and such research, like all modern scientific research, is theoretical as well as empirical.

2) Almost from its start, modern medicine has made increasing use of basic research, particularly physics, chemistry, anatomy, and physiology, as well as of statistics and engineering, whereas premodern medicine did not.

3) From the mid-nineteenth century, medicine used not only observational data but also experimental, demographic, and epidemiological ones.

4) From the beginning of the twentieth century, routine medical examinations have involved biochemical, bacteriological, parasitological, and other analyses.

5) Since the mid-nineteenth century, *randomized controlled studies* have been conducted, and some of them have been made on samples constituted by thousands of individuals.

6) From about 1800, medics have used not only the five senses, but also precision observation and measurement instruments. These are not

only more precise than the naked senses, they also reach imperceptible things, such as capillaries and bacteria, as well as imperceptible processes, such as tumor growth and chemical reactions.

7) Modern medicine resorts to data not only to evaluate treatments but also to evaluate hypotheses in the lab. Moreover, there is a consensus that untestable hypotheses have no room in medicine, and that the hypotheses on mechanisms of action are the deepest and therefore the most interesting and promising, since mechanisms, if known, can be tampered with.

In short, all medicines proper have been evidence-based, but only from the mid-sixteenth century on, and particularly since about 1800, medicine has made intensive use of the scientific method, the basic sciences, and instrumentation, to which we owe, among others, the X-ray machine (Röntgen in 1895), radioisotopes, and brain-imaging devices, all of which would be unthinkable without atomic and nuclear physics.

And the intense search for disease mechanisms did not start vigorously and systematically until Rudolf Virchow proposed his hypothesis that all diseases originate in abnormal changes within cells. Until then, most medics had remained satisfied with meticulous descriptions — preferably of morgue material. Worse, the positivists — the only philosophers who interacted with scientists at the time — warned against attempts to explain anything: descriptivism prevailed. Only a few researchers dared ask questions of the form *How does it work?*, which invite digging for mechanisms beneath appearances.

The disease-mechanism chasers were the ones who made many unexpected if frightening findings and invented ingenious artifacts. (Note the distinction, essential to philosophical realism, between discovering what there is and inventing what might be done.) It suffices to recall the following discoveries: of viruses, antibodies, oncogenes, allergies, stress, superbugs, and AIDS.

As for some of the inventions that changed the face of medicine, and even the way we live in the advanced countries, recall the randomized controlled experiment; a whole raft of vaccines and another of antibiotics; the designer drugs, such as the contraceptive pill and psychotropic and antihypertensive drugs; chemotherapy, laparoscopy, and organ transplant;

and such feats of medical physics and engineering as stents and neural prostheses. Compare these achievements in one century with two millennia of stagnation in traditional medicine.

To better appreciate the distance between modern and ancient medicine, suffice it to recall that the latter did not have any of the instruments that any contemporary medic and nurse use: the wristwatch, thermometer, stethoscope, and blood pressure gauge. Galileo measured time intervals using his own pulse, because the pocket watch came much later. Until then, the few medics who took the pulse — those in "the pulse school" — paid attention to its firmness, regularity, and "quality" (whatever this meant), but not to its rate. (The general notion of a rate was exactified much later by Newton's concept of a fluxion, or time derivative.) Before 1867, when Thomas Allbutt invented the first practical medical thermometer, a physician could feel with his hands whether his patient was feverish, but not whether her temperature had passed the critical values of 37°C or 42°C. And before 1896, when Scipione Riva-Rocci invented the first practical sphygmomanometer, nobody measured blood pressures. In short, measurement of the four vital signs was neither accurate nor popular much before the twentieth century.

Furthermore, the classical medics could know nothing of leukocyte count or metabolic rate, of lung caverns or cardiovascular accidents. Except in very obvious cases, such as flesh wounds and bone fractures, the ancient and medieval medics had to proceed in the dark; they were forced to practice what nowadays is called *holistic medicine*, which we repute as a variety of medical quackery. And their primitive knowledge led them frequently to ridiculous and barbaric procedures, such as bloodletting to treat the lesions caused on slaves by shackles and chains.

Still, modern medicine did not replace the whole of traditional medicine, but was the product of the convergence of Hippocratic–Galenic medicine with anatomy (Vesalius), physiology (Harvey), mechanics (Borelli), chemistry (van Helmont), and microscopy (Leeuwenhoek). Modern anatomy was born the same year 1543 as when Copernicus' heliocentric model of the solar system was published. Indeed, that was the publication date of the earliest modern anatomical atlas, *De humani corporis fabrica*, by the Flemish surgeon Andreas Vesalius, which contained stunning illustrations, as beautiful as they were precise. That book resulted from one more fusion: that of science with art. It was also ideologically important, in that it restored the pagan admiration for the beauty of the human body, which Christianity had regarded as base and deserving punishment.

True, half a century earlier, Leonardo da Vinci had made hundreds of realistic anatomical drawings, but only in 1900 had a sample of that clandestine work been published. (It was then found that the author had drawn the heart from that of monkeys.) Thus, Leonardo preceded Vesalius by half a century but, because of censorship, he was not Vesalius' precursor. And of course, the ancient Egyptian embalmers had much empirical knowledge of the viscera, but knew almost nothing about their functions. For example, the only organ they did not keep in their canopic vases was the brain, because they believed that its function was to segregate mucus. In any event, their artisanal knowledge was not incorporated into medicine, a discipline and profession of a superior social class, that of scribes.

The history of anatomy confutes Karl Popper's thesis (1963) that scientific advances are not born either from observations or from experiments, but from myths and criticisms of the latter. Actually, neither Hippocrates nor Galen gained celebrity for shooting down myths, nor for replacing them with falsifiable hypotheses; we remember them with admiration and gratitude for having conducted meticulous if rather superficial observations that generated new knowledge and, in particular, stimulated the generation of interesting hypotheses, such as that of nature's healing power.

From the start, science has advanced through observation and hypothesis, action and constructive criticism, all of which have happened within a philosophical matrix. This matrix was constituted by some principles that stimulated research, such as those of the reality and knowability of the world around the explorer. We shall return in Chapter 10 to this important if neglected topic.

Neither data nor laws suffice for understanding what has been observed, measured, or computed; to understand what is going on in a thing we must seek to explain the facts in question. And explaining, in contrast to describing, involves conjecturing or exhibiting mechanisms, most of which are imperceptible, e.g., because they are too small or too big. And that, trying to explain through mechanisms, is what Vesalius' successors did after his time; that is, from 1543 on, they built physiology, biophysics, biochemistry, scientific surgery, and epidemiology. Let us recall a few milestones.

Ambroise Paré (1546) applied Vesalius' anatomical findings to surgery; William Harvey (1628) suggested that the heart works like a hydraulic pump that forces blood to circulate around the cardiovascular system, which, counter to intuition, includes the lungs; the Epicurean (materialist) Girolamo Fracastoro (1646) described syphilis and proposed the hypothesis that this and other diseases occur through the transmission of microorganisms, which explains most of the serious diseases between the birth of civilization and the mid-twentieth century; Jan Baptista van Helmont (1648) affirmed that digestion is a chemical process; Thomas Wharton (1656) described glands; John Graunt (1662) published one of the earliest mortality tables; in 1665 Robert Hooke discovered the cell, and Marcello Malpighi the capillaries, on top of which he asserted that the body is a machine, blatant heresy to the ruling vitalism; Antony Leeuwenhoek (1676) discovered bacteria, but it will take a while to learn that there are 10 of them for every cell in our body; René Descartes (1664) and Gian Alfonso Borelli (1680) explained the muscular–skeleton system in terms of tubes, levers, pulleys, and bellows; and Thomas Sydenham described measles and scarlet fever (1676), and treated anemia with iron compounds.

In short, during the seventeenth century, medicine discarded the last remnants of religion and magic, and embraced wholeheartedly the materialist worldview, along with the rationalist and empiricist epistemology guiding the Scientific Revolution that put its stamp on the century.

As we have just seen, physics and chemistry made a decisive contribution to the birth and development of modern medicine. Unsurprisingly, the first reductionist programs were proposed during that period: those of the above-mentioned iatrophysicists and iatrochemists, as well as of the wondrous Paracelsus, a blend of imaginative scientist and charlatan. They are the ancestors of contemporary biophysics, biochemistry, and molecular biology. They accounted for some of the physical and chemical aspects of life, and discarded the vitalism of the Aristotelians. Being radical reductionists, they refused to admit that living beings possess properties that their constituents lack — a weakness that explained the persistence of vitalism until the beginning of the twentieth century.

One may smile at these reductionist essays. But it would be silly to deny their boldness and to fail to admit that, every time we take a blood pressure reading, we pay homage to the iatrophysicists, and every time we take a pill, we justify the iatrochemists.

I submit that modern biology and medicine are *emergentist materialist* rather than either vitalist or reductionist. That is, those disciplines not only regard organisms as systems endowed with physical and chemical properties, but also with typically biological properties. Metabolism, cell division, robustness, the ability to evaluate some stimuli as beneficial and others as harmless, and descent from abiotic system, are among those emergent properties (Bunge 1979; Mahner & Bunge 1997).

Robustness or resilience — the ability to recover from environmental attacks — is admirable but not mysterious; cybernetics explained it "mechanistically" in the mid-twentieth century in terms of negative feedback. This consists in that part of the output of a system feeds back into it, to weaken the intensity of the input, thus creating the illusion of goal-seeking. (In the simplest case, the process is described by this formula for the rate of change dX/dt of a property X: "$dX/dt = a - bX$.")

Another peculiarity of organisms is that they are born and they die, so that age is an important property of theirs. This is why some dynamical theories in biology and medicine contain two time variables: public and private, or common to everything, and biological time or age.

Most scientists and some philosophers have been familiar with emergence since George Lewes — George Eliot's companion — described it in 1874 (see Blitz 1992). However, molecular biology, born in 1953, revived for a while the reductionist dream (or nightmare), this time in the form of DNAism. This is the myth that everything biotic is purely molecular and, more specifically, reducible to DNA — hence without *bios*. Richard Dawkins, a major player in the molecular reductionism movement, put it clearly: the very existence of organisms is paradoxical, for they would be nothing but funnels for transmitting DNA from one generation (of what if not organisms) to the next.

If such a radical version of reductionism were true, we would have to assume either that anxiety or depression do not exist, or that even viruses, which are clumps of DNA, can get anxious or depressed. Fortunately, psychiatry, though far from perfect, does not explain mental diseases in purely molecular terms, any more than botanists explain the life of plants by studying only their seeds. In the eye of the radical reductionist, the world is as flat as a pancake, so that emergence is either nonexistent or mysterious. But the ubiquity of emergence and the corresponding variety of the sciences suggests a different metaphor — that of the layered cake.

Consequently, to account for complex facts, we must often combine top-down explanations with bottom-up ones. This is the case of the chronic psychological stress caused by macrosocial facts such as war, unemployment, or gender discrimination. They may affect the chromosomes, a harm which in turn elicits systemic ailments such as diabetes and cardiovascular disease, with the aggregate social consequences of decreased productivity and increased burden on the sanitary system (e.g., Nestler 2012). (See Figure 2.1.)

To resume our sketchy story of medicine, physicalism and chemism were primitive but perhaps unavoidable phases of materialist philosophy, biology, and medicine. And it is no accident that iatrophysics and iatro-chemistry, along with their corresponding therapies, developed at about the same time as that of modern machinery, in particular the steam engine. Fully modern man, born at the time of the American and French Revolutions, tends to believe that machines, not angels or demons, are power sources.

L'homme machine (1747), the banned work of the physician and phi-losopher Julien Offray de La Mettrie, was the popular mechanistic mani-festo of the French Enlightenment — not of the Renaissance or the Scientific Revolution, let alone that of the Romantic reaction or that of postmodernity. La Mettrie had learned the "mechanical method" from its champion, Herman Boerhaaven — the botanist, chemist, and eminent professor of medicine at Leiden University.

A few years later, Paul-Henri Thiry, Baron d'Holbach, the great systemic materialist mentioned earlier, studied at the same university — the only one

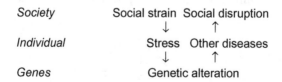

Fig. 2.1. A top-down process intertwined with a bottom-up one. The genetic change occurring in the last link of the downward chain may consist in the shortening of telomeres or in the methylation of DNA — a heresy before the emergence of epigenetics only five years ago. (See also Figure 2.2.)

in the world where basic science was being done and taught at the time. D'Holbach interacted with La Mettrie as well as with other members of the French Enlightenment, who in turn interacted with those of the progressive intellectual of the time (see Blom 2010).

The medical establishment was so entrenched, that it took half a century for the French Enlightenment to make an impact on medicine. But this impact was so strong that it affected biomedical research, the practice of medicine, and public health care. Suffice it to recall the French hospitals and asylums at the beginning of the nineteenth century, as well as the German and Austrian ones half a century later. All of them were research centers, and their patients were given the best medical assistance. However, let us return to the mechanistic conception of the organism.

Except for the marginal school of artificial life in Santa Fe, USA, whose members believe that their computer models are alive, no one believes that organisms are machines, if only because machines, unlike living things, are designed. We believe even less in the vitalist and spiritualist views of life, because we know that organisms are very sensitive to physical and chemical stimuli. Moreover, we know that humans occupy all the levels of organization. Indeed, although our constituents are physico-chemical, we are alive for a while, we belong to various social organizations, and our upbringing, mental life, and social activities make us artificial, to the point that our prefrontal cortex exerts a cognitive control over our behavior, which allows us to live together as well as to compete. (See Figure 2.2.)

The preceding view conflicts with the popular view that medicine is reductionist, just because it is based on physics and chemistry. That opinion is false, because all medics know that their patients are capable of undergoing processes, such as those of taking initiatives, inventing problems, feeling, planning, and influencing other people, that not even the

ARTIFACTS
SOCIETY
INTELLIGENT LIFE
LIFE
CHEMISM
PHYSICAL LEVEL

Fig. 2.2. The six main levels of reality.

smartest computer can do. To repeat: *we exist on several levels*. Hence, the physician who forgets this point won't understand that obesity, hypertension, stress, addictions, and many other disabling conditions are largely due to social inadaptations, wrong decisions, or harmful social impacts.

That is why many medical treatments involve educating the patient or helping her alter her social environment. For example, thanks to the reform instituted by Philippe Pinel (1794), the individuals diagnosed as schizophrenics, who used to be confined or even beaten up, were promoted to the category of sick poople, and are now treated with psychopharmaceutical drugs. The drug addicts, who used to be regarded as perverts or delinquents, are now being treated as mental patients capable of being re-educated. And of course the homosexuals, who used to be persecuted, segregated, or even subjected to cruel treatments, have been demedicalized. In sum, contemporary medicine is neither reductionistic nor inhumane.

The preceding characterization of the rise of modern medicine is bound to disappoint the admirers of Michel Foucault (1963), who is currently the most cited scholar in the humanities. For example, Foucault claimed that modern medicine is empiricist to the point of rejecting theory and philosophy, whereas we have emphasized the role of hypothesis in biomedical research and practice, as well as the strong impact of philosophy on the discipline since antiquity. Foucault also claimed that the crucial difference between modern and traditional medicine is linguistic, whereas our account has focused on biological discoveries, such as Harvey's, medical inventions such as the vaccines, and philosophical presuppositions such as rationality, realism, and materialism. Lastly, whereas Foucault mentioned only Frenchmen, we, following the professional historians of medicine, have mentioned scientists and physicians from half a dozen European countries. A relativist would say that the choice among alternative historical and medical "narratives" is just a matter of taste, convention, or politics. They reason like Groucho Marx when he said, "Those are my principles. If you don't like them, I have got others." Let the reader choose.

2.2 From the Enlightenment to Experimental Medicine

During the eighteenth century, the biomedical investigators kept advancing in the direction suggested by their precursors in the previous century.

One of the many accomplishments of the *Siècle des Lumières* was the discovery that eating citrus fruits prevents scurvy. This was the unexpected finding of James Lind (1753), the physician with the British navy who subjected to experimental test what he had been told about the beneficial effect of lime juice, rich in what two centuries later would be identified with vitamin C. His seems to have been the massive medical experiment, comparable in scale only to the trial performed in Puerto Rico in 1956 to test the effectiveness of the first oral contraceptive.

Lind's discovery did not remain confined to the medical community, but motivated the British government to plant a large number of lime trees in the island of Cyprus for the use of the British navy. This was the first large agricultural and medical enterprise, as well as an extraordinary case of convergence of medico-military experience, scientific experiment, and imperialism.

In 1778, John Hunter published the first treatise of scientific dentistry, and shortly thereafter studied inflammation and experimented with gonorrhea on himself. When his disciple Edward Jenner told him that he "thought" that the individuals who had suffered cowpox remained immunized against smallpox, Hunter famously replied, "Don't think, Jenner. Experiment!" Jenner performed the experiment, and in 1798 invented the smallpox vaccine.

Some of the traditional medical schools, in particular the Ayurvedic and the Ottoman ones, knew the vaccination principle, but applied it only sporadically and on a very small scale. Even nowadays, compulsory vaccination is resisted by fanatics of natural products and by some religious and political sects. In 1885, when an outbreak of smallpox appeared in Montreal, it struck only the French Canadians, who defied the quarantine and the vaccination decreed by the sanitary authority. They opposed these measures by force for believing what the Catholic Church told them, that the epidemic was punishment for their sins, and what the French Canadian nationalists claimed, that it was an Anglo conspiracy (Bliss 2011). Similarly, in 2012, a group of health care workers who were inoculating Afghan children against polio, were murdered by Taliban fanatics, who claimed that vaccination was a Western conspiracy.

Let us now go back to the nineteenth century, which the famous philosopher José Ortega y Gasset called "stupid." That century was that of the triumph of modernity announced by the French Enlightenment. In fact, it produced modern scientific medicine, as well as effective and massive sanitary assistance. It also gave us statistics, evolutionary biology, experimental medicine, neuroscience, and the first glimmer of biological psychiatry, as well as field physics, atomic chemistry, the discovery of the electron, X-rays and radioactivity, plus bacteriology, biochemical pharmacology as well as universal suffrage, trade unionism, cooperativism, socialism, and the embryo of the welfare state, which has accomplished so much for public health.

Suffice it to remember Mary Shelley's Frankenstein (1818), the imaginary lab-made man; the first synthesis of an "organic" product, urea (Wöhler in 1828); the reductionist program in biology and medicine (1847); the *Communist Manifesto* (1848); and, above all, Darwinism (1859), or evolutionary biology, which not only asserted the evolution of all biospecies, but also explained that it had occurred through *natural* selection — something no religion could admit.

Any of these novelties should have drawn the attention of the philosophers of the time, because they called for a renewal of ontology, epistemology, and social philosophy. But they passed unnoticed to the vast majority of them. In fact, most philosophy professors remained shackled to the idealist philosophies of Kant or Hegel; the positivists, following the phenomenalism of Hume and Kant, refused to admit the existence of atoms and fields; and the Marxists admired more Hegel's cryptic formulas than Newton's or Maxwell's clarities. In short, most philosophers were stuck in the scholastic tradition of commentary and criticism. The only exception was the Leibnizian Bernhard Bolzano, mathematician and philosopher, but he influenced no one but Georg Cantor, the father of set theory, then an arcane field.

The midwife of the extraordinary scientific development of the nineteenth century was not the university philosophy, but the worldview of the radical wing of the French Enlightenment — the secular, rationalist, materialist, realist, scientistic, and humanist conception sketched by d'Holbach, Helvétius, Diderot, La Mettrie, Condorcet, and their friends, as well as other collaborators of the colossal *Encyclopédie*. This work exalted not only science but also engineering and the crafts, which had been ignored or even despised by the writers, jurists, and philosophers, who

Table 2.1. Main features of transformations championed by the radical wing of the French Enlightenment.

Aspect	Transformation
Logical	Dogmatism → Rationalism.
Ontological	Idealism → Materialism.
Epistemological	Empiricism → Scientism.
Praxiological	Primacy of contemplation → Primacy of action.
Ethical	Deontology → Humanism, egalitarianism, utilitarianism.
Political	Constitutional monarchism → Democracy.

constituted the bulk of the intelligentsia. The re-evaluation of technology and craftsmanship had an impact on medicine, a field where only surgeons used their hands. Indeed, it was only in the next century that medics began to invent instruments, starting with the stethoscope (1816), which since then has been the badge of the medical profession. As well, surgeons were promoted; they were allowed to move from the guild of barbers to that of medics.

Table 2.1 summarizes the characteristics of the philosophy created by the radical wing of the French Enlightenment. This movement is less known today than the Scottish Enlightenment, which was equally enthusiastic over rationality and secularism but discarded ontology (metaphysics), held a timid epistemology (phenomenalism), and was politically conservative. These differences explain why the French Enlightenment had a much stronger influence on science and society than the Scottish one. Where the Scots were content to get rid of religion, the French wished to replace it with science, as well as to rebuild society along rational and humane lines. The French, not the Scots, inspired the American and the French Revolutions, and modern medicine came of age in Paris, not Edinburgh.

The same enlightened philosophy also inspired the ambitious reductonist program in the mid-nineteenth century. This program not only repudiated the remains of vitalism and of *Naturphilosophie* (Goethe, Hegel, Schelling, and Oken), but it also attempted to reduce biology to physics and chemistry, the way that the iatrophysicists and iatrochemists of the seventeenth century had tried. The new reductionist program was embraced not only by the "vulgar (or mechanistic) materialists": the popular writers Büchner, Vogt, and Moleschott. It was also proclaimed by the 1847 *Manifesto* signed by some of the most respected biomedical researchers of the time: Hermann von Helmholtz, Emil du Bois-Reymond, Karl Ludwig, and Ernst Brücke. However, let us go back to 1800.

Nineteenth-century biomedical research started wih medical pathology, which discovered the anatomical traces that many diseases and toxics leave. But what escaped those diligent and meticulous pathologists was nearly as interesting as what they found. For instance, they could not possibly have found the irreversible lesions caused by epileptic seizures, much less by deep and prolonged depressions. These lesions escaped them not only because the electron microscope was produced only a century later, but also because of the predominance of psychoneural dualism, which was embraced not only by the great psychiatrist Hughlins Jackson, one of Freud's heroes, but even the eminent neuroscientists Charles Sherrington (synapse), Wilder Penfield (mental events caused by electrical stimulation of the cortex), and Roger Sperry (split brain), all of whom contributed so much to the explanation of the mental by the neural — they were psychoneural dualists.

The same dualism is inherent in the functionalist (in particular computerist) speculative psychology shared by most philosophers of mind. This antiquated view of mind discourages the search for the so-called neural "substrates" (or "correlates") of mental disorders, hence it is a severe obstacle to their biological treatment.

A different bias delayed the discovery of the thin nerves linking the cerebral cortex to the condensed immune system. Who but a dualist could believe the old-wives' tales about the therapeutic effects of prayer or of shamanic ceremonies? And yet, those neural links exist, and they help explain the successes of psycho-neuro-endocrino-immuno-pharmacology. We will reurn to this in Chapter 7.

Until the mid-nineteenth century, biomedical research had been primarily observational with heavy emphasis on the study of dead bodies. Claude Bernard changed that nearly overnight, when he performed the earliest controlled physiological experiments on live animals, and published his *Introduction à l'étude de la médecine expérimentale* (1865). This book, which had an extraordinary diffusion, became a classic of basic science and philosophy of science. (Its title is somewhat misleading, because it deals with experiments in physiology not in medicine.) In it Bernard explained, among things, why experiment trumps observation: because it involves the control of variables and therefore the possibility of finding and testing causal hypotheses.

We also owe to Bernard his capital hypothesis, which Walter Cannon confirmed and expanded on half a century later, that the organism, far from being a passive toy of its environment, adapts actively to it, as it maintains a fairly constant internal milieu, which endows it with a certain autonomy. This limited autonomy is a peculiarity of organisms, in contradistinction to physico-chemical systems.

It is to be noted that the experimental subjects ("animal models") that Bernard and others used were frogs, rabbits, dogs, cats, monkeys, and other creatures, and that genetics studies in bacteria, fruit flies, and worms concern biological processes so basic that they also occur in humans. This practice of using "animal models," which goes back to Galen, tacitly presupposes the heterodox thesis, proposed by Buffon and reinvented a century later by Charles Darwin, of the *unity of life* — that all living beings are interrelated. For example, we share the *Hox* genes with fruit flies, worms, and other lowly organisms.

This kinship is genuine and deep, not mere analogy, and it consists in having more or less remote common ancestors. This kinship makes it possible for drugs to be tried out on guinea pigs and other animals before using humans. Besides, evolutionary biology has taught us that some of our biological defects, such as flat feet, chronic back pain, and troublesome wisdom teeth, are taxes we have to pay for having parted company with the great apes some six million years ago.

In short, modern medicine has developed in close interaction with the basic sciences. But in many cases, it has had to contend with the ruling religions and philosophies. A recent conflict between medicine and organized religion was abused by the use of stem cells from miscarriages and abortions; a second, far more serious conflict, was originated from the religious and political ban on contraceptives and abortions. The former prohibition has slowed down the design and trial of some therapies. The second ban has contributed to the spread of AIDS, as well as to the increase in the number of neglected or even abandoned children, as well as of women with truncated studies and careers.

As for the harmful effect of certain philosophies on medicine, it suffices to recall the views that all diseases are either iatrogenic or social conventions, and the schools in clinical psychology and psychiatry that persist in ignoring the brain. A particularly effective offender has been the functionalist view of the mind, that usually comes along with the opinion that everything mental is only information processing, hence equally realizable in brains, computers, or even immaterial souls. This philosophical school ignores neuroscience and discourages experiment, while encouraging wild speculation, like that of the self-styled evolutionary psychologists. By the same token, these fantasists have retarded the development of effective psychiatric treatments.

2.3 The Systemic Approach

One of the peculiarities of contemporary medicine is that it is composed of dozens of specialties, from traumatology to psychiatry. That is, medicine is a *multidiscipline*. However, every one of its branches is more or less strongly linked to the others. For example, modern traumatology, unlike the ancient crafts of bone-setting and amputation, makes intensive use of anatomy and physiology. By contrast, the primitive and archaic medicines, as well as the so-called alternative medicines, are isolated bodies of belief and practice. In particular, they are not based on science and they do not examine their own philosophical presuppositions.

That the human body is a system is a comparatively recent discovery. How do we find out whether two or more organs are part of a system? By looking for bonds among them and, once found, by severing such links. Let us briefly recall a couple of daring and fruitful experiments of that kind, centered in diabetes — a serious, incurable, and systemic (whole-body) disease that is on the rise around the world. In 1887, Oskar Minkowski discovered that the pancreas makes insulin and that, when deprived of its pancreas, an animal becomes severely diabetic and dies, because it does not produce the insulin required to metabolize sugar, the body's fuel. Much later, it was found that the hypophysis, or pituitary gland, is the master internal gland — it secretes nine hormones that regulate homeostasis, metabolism, growth, and more.

Nearly one century ago, the Argentine physiologist Bernardo A. Houssay made a surprising discovery in faraway Buenos Aires: that an animal deprived of its pituitary gland becomes hypoglycemic when injected with a small amount of insulin. Since the latter is secreted by the pancreas, there had to be an intimate pituitary–pancreas connection. It was natural to ask what would happen if this connection were severed. So, in 1929, Houssay and colleagues performed an experiment whereby the pituitary gland was ablated from a dog that had been deprived of its pancreas. Surely, something dramatic had to happen after two such radical surgeries. And so it did: the dog recovered unexpectedly from diabetes, although it did not survive long. For once, two wrongs made a right.

An important discovery had been made, that the pancreas and the pituitary, though far from each other, are components of a single system, the endocrine one. Consequently, endocrinology was transformed overnight, from the study of individual internal glands into the multidisciplinary science of the endocrine system — another triumph of systemism. At about the same time, in Montreal, Hans Selye was crafting another synthesis: that of endocrinology and immunology. The two discoveries in basic science had impacts on medicine, the former on the management of diabetes and the latter on that of stress.

A union of scientific or medical disciplines is not a mere juxtaposition, but a cohesive synthesis, an "organic whole" or *system*. And the cement that joins the constituents of any such system is constituted by material bridges and their conceptual counterparts, such as the hypothesis that mental diseases are brain disorders — whence biology is highly relevant to psychiatry, and the mental patients should not be segregated from the others.

In other words, modern medicine is not an aggregate but a system of disciplines, and its practitioners interact with one another because each of them knows a part of the same whole. In turn, this epistemic unity is due to the fact that all the medical specialties deal with the same thing: the patient, an animal very much like other animals, except for its exceptionally evolved brain and social life. This is why René Dubos (1959), in an influential book, emphasized that the patient should be treated as a totality and as inserted in his social milieu.

As with other fields, in medicine it is systems all the way, from molecule to cell to organ to whole organism to nature to society. This is why one sees, with increasing frequency, references to *systemic biology* (e.g., Rigoutsos & Stephanopoulos 2007; Loscalzo & Barabasi 2011). And contemporary medicine encourages us to look for

biosystems (e.g., nervous, endocrine, and neuro-endocrino-immune),
epistemic systems (e.g., biology, medicine, and medical humanities), and
sociosystems (e.g., hospital, medical community, market, and state).

We may distinguish systems of various genera: *concrete* or material in a broad sense (e.g., cells and societies), *conceptual* or fictitious (e.g., classifications and theories), *semiotic* or meaningful (e.g., texts and diagrams), and *technological* (e.g., sphygmomanometers and ambulances).

In turn, a concrete system σ is an object characterizable by the following traits:

Composition of σ = Set of all the parts of σ.
Immediate environment of σ = Set of all the entities, different from σ, that may interact with σ.
Structure of σ = Set of the relations among the parts of σ (endostructure), and among these and the environment of σ (exostructure).
Mechanism of σ = Process(es) peculiar to σ, or what makes σ tick.

Notice that we distinguish systems from their models, if only because any given system may be represented by different models. The above model holds for concrete (material) systems, whether natural or social. If a system is either conceptual or semiotic, the last component of the above quadruple must be deleted, because such systems do not change by themselves nor, consequently, do they have mechanisms.

Individualists have no use for systems; they are only interested in their constituents, and consequently they miss the systemic or emergent properties, such as those of being alive or dead, and in good or bad health. Holists, by contrast, reject analysis and minimize, or even deny, the role of the individual. Systemism, the alternative to both individualism and holism, keeps the valid theses of each of them, that there is no whole without parts, and that some wholes (the "organic" ones or systems) have global properties that their parts lack. Systemism is thus a synthesis of individualism and holism.

In particular, the good physician is a systemist: she prefers syndromes to isolated symptoms, places the body in its environment, and takes into account all the relevant levels of organization of matter, from the physical to the social. Indeed, she will tacitly embrace the following principles:

1) *The human being is a system of subsystems.* Medical lesson: Every reasonably complete medical examination will look at the whole body and its environment, and will focus on its critical mechanisms, with a view to repair the defective ones;

2) *All the subsystems of the human body are interconnected,* either directly (by tissues) or indirectly (through blood and hormones). Example: the oto-rhyno-laringeal system. Medical moral: Every treatment, however local, has distal effects, some of which are likely to be adverse, which is why all treatments are perfectible but none will ever be perfect;

3) *Every disease consists of a dysfunction of one or more organs,* and every chronic sickness is concomitant with other disorders (comorbidities). Medical lesson: Every medical treatment must seek the recovery of the normal functions of the affected parts, as well as the protection of the others;

4) *Mental health is brain health,* and consequently a part of total health. Medical moral: Do not neglect the possible mental effects (e.g., anxiety and depression) of chronic diseases and drastic treatments;

5) *Individual well-being and social condition are closely linked*; in particular, poverty and oppression breed morbidity. Medical lesson: The pursuit of personal well-being includes the control over the environment, in particular of factors such as environmental pollution, crowding, as well as work safety and security (see Bunge 2012b);

6) Given the complexity of humans and their social enviroment, physicians should *avoid sectoral (or sectional) thinking,* that which (a) detaches and isolates things, properties, and processes that in fact go together; (b) tends to "anchor" in first impressions, data, or conjectures (see Kahneman 2011); and (c) worsens the balkanization of medicine instead of building interdisciplinary bridges; and

7) *One-size-fits-all explanations must be distrusted* in medicine as much as in social science. For example, we still do not know for sure why one can get fat, or why obesity is increasing worldwide. Several explanations have been proposed: inborn predisposition, overeating, excess

carbohydrate ingestion, and sedentarism. Perhaps the correct answer is: all of the preceding.

The emergence of the systemic approach in biology and medicine in modern times confirms the *systemic philosophy* that Paul-Henri Thiry, Baron d'Holbach (1966) introduced in 1770. This eminent and prolific polymath and political dissident was a conspicuous collaborator of the famous *Encyclopédie* (1751–1772) edited by Denis Diderot, initially jointly with Jean le Rond d'Alembert. With very few exceptions, contemporary philosophers have ignored the very concept of a system, which is characteristic of modern science and technology, or they have mistaken it for that of an unanalyzable whole used by the holistic philosophers from Aristotle to Hegel.

Systemism may be summarized in the formula "Every existent is either a system or part of a system." This postulate should not be mistaken for Hegel's *Das Wahre ist das Ganze* ("The truth is the whole"). This cryptic metaphysical formula is typical of holism, which opposes both individualism and d'Holbach's systemic materialism.

Holism joins but confuses; individualism distinguishes but detaches; only systemism joins without confusing. For example, from a systemic perspective, a patient is an extremely complex system immersed in the social system, and medicine is a multidiscipline that interacts with other fields of knowledge and action that interact with other fields of knowledge and action. Moreover, in this perspective, medicine looks not like a department store, but like a vast mansion without partitions — the way the great intellectual leaders of the discipline, like Rudolf Virchow, Claude Bernard, William Osler, and Lewis Thomas, saw it. This, the systemic approach, is the best prescription against hyperspecialization, that is at variance with the unity of the human body. Clearly, a medicine-friendly philosophy will favor systemism.

Coda

Modern medicine developed from around 1550 on the basis of the biological sciences, and since 1850 it has been advancing very rapidly thanks to the modernization of the universities as well as the development of biochemistry and pharmacology. The engine of this prodigious progress of medicine has been scientific research. Without it, medicine would still be mired in myth and common sense.

Consider, for instance, the belief that sedentarism is bad for the heart. This belief seems so obvious, that it was not put to the test until very recently. The finding of a six-year longitudinal study involving 276 individuals of both sexes between the ages of 18 and 65 (Saunders *et al.* 2013) is that sedentary behavior, while it increases waist circumference, does not increase cardiometabolic risk. Only scientists can get away with "crazy" ideas, to the point that the best science journals regularly reject submissions that are not "crazy" (original) enough. The whole history of science is a sequence of "crazy" ideas, like that of acquired immunity, and "crazy" tools, like the brain-imaging ones.

By the mid-twentieth century, most of the bacterial infections, in particular tuberculosis and the venereal diseases, could be cured. There were also vaccines to prevent most of the infectious diseases, particularly those that struck the members of this writer's cohort, except in the poor countries, where they still thrive. These great advances resulted from the combination of biomedical research and enlightened sanitary policies.

The traits of the medical advances that should have drawn the attention of philosophers are the adoption of scientism and the corresponding rejection of antiscience and pseudoscience; the close union of medicine with the so-called hard sciences; the adoption of the experimental method, in particular the randomized controlled trial; the search for mechanisms of action, in particular etiologies; and the tacit admission of emergentist and systemic materialism.

However, the philosopher should also take note of the persistence of many absurd and harmful medical superstitions, in particular those parading as "alternative and complementary" medicines (recall Section 1.3). And if she is socially responsible, she will help analyze and expose such fossils, not only in professional journals, but also in the mass media.

CHAPTER 3

DISEASE

3.1 Symptom: Feeling Unwell

Had we been well designed, that is, with knowledge, intelligence, imagination, and foresight, and if our body were as wise as has often been said,
we would never get sick except through accident. But in fact we do get
sick once in a while, and our ancestors used to catch serious diseases more
often than we do, sometimes through infections and at other times because
of malnutrition, poor hygiene, or bad lifestyles, or else injury due to war
or to other acts of collective violence.

The paleoanthropologists inform us that the bipedal posture brought
diseases that we are still suffering from, such as back pain and flat feet, as
well as proneness to fractures of various kinds. It is also known that our
primitive ancestors suffered from chronic diseases such as arthritis, and that
their lifespans were far shorter than ours. All that changed some 15,000
years ago with the Neolithic Revolution, characterized by the emergence
of agriculture, and eventually irrigation and granaries. This new kind of
labor solved the problem of food scarcity and irregularity, but, like nearly
all advances, agriculture had its dark side.

Archaeology and historical demography inform us that the Neolithic
Revolution was accompanied by a population explosion and urbanization.
In turn, the latter involved crowding and pollution, which in turn favored
the propagation of infectious diseases, which until very recently claimed
more victims than the non-communicable ones, such as heart disease, cancer, and stroke. Many infectious diseases, such as smallpox, measles, diphtheria, typhoid fever, AIDS, and even influenza, were originally zoonoses,
that is, animal diseases (see, e.g., Diamond 1997: 206 ff). This was the stiff
price paid for animal domestication. Nor was it the only price that the
huge Neolithic leap exacted.

As many more cereals than wild plants were consumed, the diet got remarkably impoverished in variety, with bad consequences for health. In particular, new diseases, typical of grain-based diets, emerged: vitamin deficiencies and tooth decay, associated with soft foods, became more prevalent. Even 10 millennia later, in Pericles' highly civilized Athens, the typical diet was imbalanced and austere, particularly by comparison with that of the Persians, according to Herodotus. No wonder the Athenians tended to regard frugality as a virtue both medical and moral.

In short, the enormous social progress of the Neolithic did not bring an overall sanitary improvement. In any event, modern man is the product of two intertwined evolutions: the biological and social ones. Hence, the very concept of evolutionary medicine (Ness & Williams 1994), as a purely biological discipline, is flawed, because we are essentially gregarious and partly artificial animals, so that our brains are socially sensitive. More on this below.

No sane person likes to feel unwell or to fully depend on others, which is why we all try to get better. There was one notable exception, though: in the early days of the Scientific Revolution, the great mathematician, physicist, and philosopher Blaise Pascal (1963: 362) wrote that God sickens us to correct us, so that good Christians accept sickness with resignation and even joy, because "the health of the body jeopardizes that of the soul."

Four centuries later, there is talk of "pain theology," and some sick people dedicate their pain to God, as if they had crafted their own sickness. Others hold the groundless Christian belief that suffering redeems. Modern legal and moral philosophers since John Howard, the great prison-reformer, hold that only education and community service can rehabilitate — a humanist view corroborated by the success of the Swedish school-prison.

The healthy person is pain-averse, and so repudiates the masochism exalted by Donatien, Marquis de Sade: the body suppresses or rejects morbid beliefs and practices, and most of the time tends to heal spontaneously. For example, fractured bones are put in plaster casts, trusting that the *vis medicatrix naturae* (healing power of nature) will join the separate parts; when pathogenic germs invade us, the immune system synthesizes antibodies that "fight" them; and when in pain, our brain produces endorphins (endogenous opiates) that alleviate pain. However, while our body synthesizes antibodies, sometimes it also produces endotoxins, and cancer cells are maintained by stem cells. Both findings spoil the metaphors of the wisdom of the body and its intelligent design. However, back to masochism.

A person who enjoys suffering is usually diagnosed as suffering from depression, and her psychiatrist attempts to cure her — alas, not always successfully. But when a woman refuses an epidural shot to alleviate birth pains because she believes in the biblical curse "Thou shalt give birth in pain!," or because she prefers the natural to the artificial, her obstetrician or midwife will have to shut up.

Evolutionary psychiatry is a secular version of the pathological opinion that in the end, sickness is good for you, for all diseases would be adaptive. In particular, depression would be advantageous because the depressive, being unable to have ambitions, would dodge risks, and would consequently enjoy an advantage over his normal competitors. (Intense suffering, social incapacitation, family disruptions, labor absenteeism, and a high rate of suicides among depressives do not count because they spoil the story.) This Panglossian fantasy originates from another one: the teleological myth that evolution is always progressive because natural selection eliminates the unfit. Demography and epidemiology confute that opinion, showing that some plagues and wars have eliminated entire well-adapted peoples along with their unique genomes (Keyfitz 1984).

Something similar may have happened with the genocides that the Old Testament attributed to Jehovah, such as the massacre of all the inhabitants of Jericho with the exception of its prostitute. In other cases, natural disasters caused large social changes. For example, the plague that killed half the population of the Byzantine Empire between 541 and the eighth century may have opened the gates for the expansion of Islam, just as the Black Plague in the fourteenth century facilitated the Renaissance by concentrating wealth, which in turn encouraged bolder commercial enterprises. By itself, biology cannot explain any of the large biosocial processes that altered the course of history, if only because it focuses on biotic processes in individuals, not on social processes. Back to health care.

The health care disciplines exist because several millennia ago some gifted individuals spotted some health problems and, instead of allowing them to follow their natural courses, decided to do something more than licking their wounds. The first thing they did was to "read" or "interpret" symptoms or subjective indicators, such as feeling nauseous or weak. The earliest healers must also have learned that some symptoms are ambiguous; for example, one may feel hot without being feverish, and sad but not depressed. That is, one must distinguish between one's feelings and what is really going on. Whoever does this will philosophize, and will even correct the great Immanuel Kant (1952: B724), who, in his *magnum opus*, held that *everything* is subjective or apparent, that the world is "a sum of appearances."

A piece of knowledge is said to be *objective* or *impersonal* if it refers exclusively to its object or referent, whereas the *subjective* or *personal* appears when the subject or individual who seeks knowledge is given priority. For example, the statement "It is cold" is objective, though not necessarily true, because it refers to the environment. By contrast, "I feel cold" refers to me, and it may be true even if the temperature of my surroundings is high.

Biology, like physics, seeks exclusively objective or impersonal truths, whereas medicine, psychology, and social science deal with subjectivity as well as with objective facts, because they deal with persons, and the way people perceive facts influence their behavior. For instance, part of the success of "alternative" medicine is that it is perceived as soft or easy on the patient.

The *object/subject* dichotomy induces the partition of the set of philosophical schools into *objectivist* (or *realist*) and *subjectivist* (or *anti-realist*). The former postulates that the subject or knower is only a tiny part of the universe, which exists by itself, whereas subjectivists claim that the universe is totally or partially in the subject's mind. All of the ancient and medieval philosophers were realists, as were Galileo and Descartes, as well as Francis Bacon and John Locke. Arguably, the Scientific Revolution would not have happened if its makers, who were only about 200 individuals distributed among six countries, had practiced introspection, as St. Augustine recommended, instead of exploring the external world.

The brilliant Christian philosopher George Berkeley (1710), who flourished at the beginning of the eighteenth century, may have been the first to argue that to be, or exist, consists in perceiving or in being perceived. He was a radical and consistent empiricist — unlike David Hume, who, for practical purposes, did not deny the autonomous existence of the external world. Many felt that Berkeley's thesis was as unassailable as it was absurd. Yet, a moment's reflection suffices to realize that it does not account for error and error-correction, which happen to be part of inquiry.

Moreover, Berkeley's thesis need not be explicitly disproved, as all exploration and transformation of reality *presupposes* its previous existence. Thus, science and technology take philosophical realism for granted; they presuppose the existence of external objects endowed with primary properties, that is, traits that those objects possess independently of our exploration (Galileo 1953: 312). The subject-dependent properties, such as taste and color, are called 'secondary qualities,' also qualia. The ontology of Berkeley and Hume is phenomenalist, in that it admits only secondary (or phenomenal) properties. Both philosophers rejected Newton's mechanics, the most advanced scientific theory of their day, because it attempted to describe and explain the motions of material bodies, which they regarded as fictitious because they possess primary qualities.

Hume (1734) did not influence natural science, but he inspired German subjective idealism; he exerted a strong influence on Kant (1787), who in turn influenced Fichte's egocentrism, Nietzsche's egoism, and Husserl's egology (or phenomenology). Unsurprisingly, none of those egocentric philosophers touched on medicine, whose aim is not self-knowledge, but inquiring about the state of health of others.

Only philosophy professors, drug addicts, and the insane can afford to "stamp out reality," as the hippies of the psychedelic 1960s wished to do. The rest of us, particularly the sick and their caregivers, had better face reality. In particular, we should conduct a "reality check," or test for either truth or effectiveness, every time a new medical conjecture or therapy is proposed. This is why laboratory and clinical trials are central to scientific medicine, by contrast with the CAMs (complementary and alternative medicines). (More on trials in Chapter 6.) Any medical doctrine that does not care for such tests, hence for both truth and effectiveness, is ineffectual and even a health hazard.

It is widely believed that positivists are realists. This belief is false, since positivism is the heir to the phenomenalism held by Berkeley, Hume, and Kant. The traditional positivists, such as Auguste Comte and John Stuart Mill, were *epistemological phenomenalists*: they held that only phenomena (appearances) can be known. By contrast, Ernst Mach was also an *ontological phenomenalist*, hence anthropocentrist: he claimed that there are only phenomena. His followers, the logical positivists, were all epistemological phenomenalists, but whereas some of them were also ontological phenomenalists, others claimed that the question of the reality of the external world was a pseudoproblem, so that philosophers had to stay neutral in the objectivism/subjectivism strife (see Ayer 1959). Neither of the two factions had anything to say about either disease or medicine.

The modern physicians have always been objectivists (realists), even while calling diseases path*ologies*, and their causes etio*logies*. Medicine was saved from subjectivism because the health caregivers take it for granted that, if someone asks for their help, it is because they are feeling unwell, not because the professional will make up a sickness for her. In other words, all caregivers take the object/subject dichotomy for granted.

To a health worker, the object/subject dichotomy splits into another two dichotomies: doctor/patient and cause/disease. While the former is unproblematic, the second dichotomy is not, and it was first analyzed by Robert Koch in the case of infectious diseases. In 1882, he stated his famous *Koch Postulates* for the attribution of a sickness to a given pathogenic organism (Porter 1997: 436). These criteria are worth recalling because they still constitute a model of rigorous medical thinking.

Koch postulated that, to prove that a given microorganism causes a certain disease, it is necessary to demonstrate in the laboratory that (a) the organism be found in every instance of the disease; (b) when extracted from the body, the germ can be produced in a pure culture maintainable over several generations; (c) the disease can be reproduced in experimental animals exposed to that culture; and (d) the organism can be retrieved from the inoculated animal and cultured again.

Obviously, Koch's criteria had to be refined in light of new discoveries, such as that every healthy organism contains pathogens in small quantities, and that some of them are viruses rather than bacteria. But this is typical of scientific hypotheses: that they are in principle corrigible. Only the founder of homeopathy and the pope are supposed to be infallible.

The object/subject dichotomy is of course the central subject of the theory of knowledge, or epistemology. Those who do not admit the said dichotomy won't appreciate the efforts of scientists and technologists to seek objective truths and avoid experimental artifacts, such as sample contamination, as well as to expose data fabrications. Only some modern authors have dared challenging the objectivism or realism inherent in scientific research. Yet, even a cursory examination suffices to show that scientific theories refer to the objects under investigation, not to their inventors, and that every careful experimental design seeks to minimize disturbances that the experimenter may cause involuntarily. This is why experimenters wash their hands, use micromanipulators, and freeze the variables that are not being measured. They are well aware of horror stories about the involuntary release of lethal pathogens into urban environments, as well as of the first recorded case of transfer of "cadaveric material" from the dissection room to the maternity ward, famously discovered in 1847 by the obstetrician Ignaz Semmelweis — a discovery that prompted a radical improvement of aseptic conditions in hospitals.

True, it is often claimed that quantum physics places the observer at the center of the world: that the universe is mental. But this thesis is false, as shown by the facts that (a) quantum theory is used to explain the nuclear reactions at the center of the Sun, which is inaccessible to observers; and (b) cosmology deals only with physical objects, so that all the talk of "participatory universe," "constructing the universe out of nothing," and of "building *its* [material things] from *bits* [information units]," are sheer myth-making (e.g., Bunge 2012a). Medics need not take such stories seriously; they are only old Berkeley's subjectivism in new garb. Only psychologists, social scientists, and psychiatrists deal with mental processes, but they treat them objectively, that is, as occurring outside the student's brain.

It is also true that, as the postmoderns emphasize, scientific research is a social process — but not a social construction or convention. Research is social only in the sense that it involves both cooperation and competition, or rather emulation. But researchers do not study themselves except in the very rare cases when they have used themselves as guinea pigs; normally they study things in their external worlds, such as molecules, animal models, or social groups. Only mathematicians and artists are exempt from the objectivity requirement.

Yet, several schools have denied the reality of diseases, or rather diseased bodies; they have claimed that health disorders are either "only in the mind" or social facts. Two notorious cases of medical nihilism are shamanism and constructivism-relativism. For instance, it is said of the Mexican peasant that he calls the veterinarian when his cow gets sick, and the shaman when his wife ails. A reason for this difference is the primitive belief that a disease of beings endowed with a soul is a mental illness caused by a spiritual agent, whether a witch or god-like creature. Nowadays, the followers of the Christian Science sect, which Mark Twain ridiculed more than a century ago, hold the same view and resort to religious ceremonies in hopes of effecting miraculous healings like those attributed to Jesus Christ.

The preceding reminds us the general methodological rule that we must know or assume something about the nature of the beast before confronting it. Whether the problem to be tackled is one of knowledge or of action, we must start by finding out whether the entity involved is worldly or otherworldly, material or spiritual, scrutable or inscrutable, and manageable or beyond our powers. That is, ontology precedes both epistemology and praxiology, because the means used to study or control an object depends on its nature.

In the case of a medical problem — that is, a problem about diseases — before tackling it we must find out or assume something about the nature of disease: whether or not it occurs objectively, whether it is a natural process or a social construction, whether biology can help understand and treat it, and so on. So, again, being precedes knowing and acting. But in turn, only research can yield detailed knowledge, which in turn is required for effective action. Thus, the medic handles, albeit usually in an implicit manner, the virtuous triangle made up of being, knowing, and doing. To reject this triangle is to perpetrate medical nihilism.

Social constructivism is one end of the medical nihilism spectrum. It holds that diseases and recoveries, far from being natural processes, are social ones. Thus, Bruno Latour (1999), a prominent member of this school, held that, contrary to the assertion of the French pathologists who examined the mummy of Ramses II (who died c. 1167 B.C.), the ancient Egyptians could not have suffered from tuberculosis, because Koch discovered the tuberculosis bacillus only three millennia later. According to Latour, the tuberculosis diagnosis in question was a clear case of interference of politics with science. Why not go the whole hog and declare that there had been no gravity before Newton?

Social constructivism-relativism is far from being the latest Parisian fashion; it is but an offshoot of Berkeley's subjectivism. It is also inherent in the Copenhagen interpretation of quantum mechanics, according to which existence is an effect of observation, so that the universe is mental rather than physical (see Bunge 1959b). Three decades later, and independently, Louis Althusser, Michel Foucault, and Jürgen Habermas supplied the political component of the "new," post-Mertonian philosophy and sociology of science and technology. They denounced both as constituting "the ideology of late capitalism," and added that scientific research is a struggle for power, not for new knowledge — but of course they offered no evidence for either thesis. So, ontological constructivism "was in the air" in the mid-twentieth century. Back now to medical constructivism.

The prophet of constructivist pathology was the Polish bacteriologist Ludwik Fleck (1979 [1935]). He won posthumous notoriety by claiming that "syphilis, as such, does not exist": that, like all "scientific facts," syphilis was a product of a "thought collective," or community of people united by a "thought style." In short, syphilis would not be a natural or even biosocial fact, but a purely cultural one. Do not ask for evidence, for this concept is unknown to the postmoderns.

The Nazis did not believe Dr. Fleck's story; they kept him alive in the concentration camp where they confined him, on the condition that he put his bacteriology to work. This he did to everyone's benefit; he advised taking prophylactic measures to prevent the spread of typhus, which is caused by bacilli that are as real as stones. That is, when the moment of truth came, the inventor of medical subjectivism faced it like a common objectivist, the way Hume faced real-life problems. (More on constructivism-relativism in Bunge 1999.)

From the constructivist perspective, there is no objective reality nor, consequently, objective truth; there would be maps without mapped territories. But common sense rebels: why believe that metabolism and blood circulation, sex and scoliosis, and dwarfism and cancer are social conventions on a par with markets and wars? After all, life precedes sociality, and there is solid archaeological evidence that diseases preceded medicine, just as the Earth preceded geography.

Social constructivism is not the only school that denies that diseases are objective natural processes. Some psychiatrists have equated mental diseases with their syndromes, thus tacitly denying what neuroscience tells us about the neural mechanisms of such disorders. (For example, a hallucination may be caused by the temporary inactivation of a group of neurons due to a local interruption of blood flow.) The history of psychiatry too is realistic, inasmuch as it shows that a given disease may be diagnosed in different ways as science evolves (Shorter 1997; Murphy 2011).

The hermeneutic or literary approach to medicine yields a similar result. In particular, Georges Canguilhem (1966), perhaps the best-known philosopher of medicine, analyzed the words 'normal' and 'abnormal,' which in medicine are usually taken as synonymous with 'healthy' and 'sick,' respectively. But the word 'normal' has a very different meaning in the social sciences and technologies, particularly in the law, where 'normal' means 'subject to norm or rule,' hence as the antonym of 'deviant.'

(In statistics, another two concepts of 'normal' occur: bell-shaped distribution, and close to the "mode" or most frequent value of the distribution, which coincides with the mean in the case of a bell-shaped one. But statistical deviance is not the same as sickness. For example, excentricity, left-handedness, synesthesia, and other uncommon traits are abnormal but not pathological, because they do not block any vital functions.)

Canguilhem confused the normative and the descriptive concepts of normality, favored the former, and concluded that diseases are social deviations, hence matters of concern in some societies and periods but not in others. The same would hold for health; it would be just a different social norm, the one we happen to prefer to its opposite here and now. Correspondingly, medicine would be a "normative project" — just like politics and the law. Thus, "normal is what results from the execution of the normative project," so that the abnormal, in particular the morbid, preexists the normal or healthy. To put it in biblical terms, "In the beginning was the morbus."

Canguilhem's extravagant views on disease and medicine should not be shrugged off without further ado, because they were adopted and developed by such influential postmodern writers as Louis Althusser, Gilles Deleuze, Jacques Derrida, and above all, Michel Foucault. Nietzsche, the prophet of postmodernism and Foucault's top hero, asserted that "truth is the deepest lie." Had he and Foucault admitted that there are truths, such as the proposition "Sexual promiscuity is unhealthy," the former might not have died from syphilis and the latter from AIDS. But then, neither of them might have attained celebrity status in an age where the absurd is worshipped even in academia.

If diseases were social conventions resulting from the "combat between knowledge and power," as Foucault (1963) held and as Roger Cooter (2007) and other admirers of his have repeated, they might be initiated and terminated by decree. But of course, medicine has taught us that diseases are natural conditions — basically physiological dysfunctions — and archaeology has found that many of them are ancient rather than recent Parisian fashions. (For more on the conflict between the normative [or constructivist] and the naturalist conceptions of disease, see Boorse 2011; Simon 2011.)

What is true is that the *understanding* of diseases as biomedical problems depends not only on knowledge but also, in part, on value judgments. For instance, until very recently, mental diseases were stigmatized. And every time a new edition of the *Diagnostic and Statistical Manual* of the American Psychiatric Association is published, a bunch of mental "disorders" are added, and a bunch of others eliminated. But nearly everyone agrees that this is only a marker of the sorry state of psychiatry.

Here is another example: in some societies, obesity, alcoholism, gambling, and snuffing cocaine were high-status symbols just because not everyone could afford them. Contemporary medicine treats them as diseases because they are objectively harmful. By contrast, in treating all diseases as social conventions or arbitrary "medicalizations," the constructivists and hermeneuticians trivialize suffering, undermine public health, and favor the vice industry.

The view we defend may be called *medical realism*. It does not hypostatize the universal "disease," but it does not deny the real existence of sick people either, regardless of social conventions. Sick individuals are real, whereas diseases are kinds, species, or types. That is, they are sets and, as such, concepts rather than words. Yet, they are not *arbitrary* groupings but *natural kinds*, just as much as the chemical and biological ones. And a natural kind is definable by a predicate representing a real property, such as "communicable," not an imaginary predicate such as "bewitched."

Moreover, not every real property defines a natural kind. For example, "feverish" defines the broad class of people suffering from fever, but this class is not a medical species, because fever is a sign of many different diseases. (Discomfort, "upset stomach," and dizziness are parallel.) Only well-defined diseases, such as gout and influenza, define medical kinds or species. (More on biospecies in Mahner & Bunge 1997.)

(Note, incidentally, the difference between a *property*, or objective trait, and an *attribute*, or *predicate*, that is attributed to something, whether with or without a reason or justification. A well-defined class is the *denotation* or *reference* of the corresponding predicate, whose *connotation* or *intension* — written with an *s*, not a *t* — is the predicate's *sense*. For example, the sense of the predicate "contagious" is "transmissible by contact," whereas its denotation is the class of all the individuals struck by a communicable disease. These individuals are real, whereas the collection they constitute is unreal. But this set is no mere fantasy, as suggested by the fact that the inclusion in it has a real correlate, namely the process of falling sick. The concepts we have just elucidated belong to the branch of philosophy called *semantics*: Bunge 1974a, 1974b.)

The medical realist does not deny the existence of imaginary patients either. Imaginary diseases come in different types:

1) The diseases imagined by the hypochondriacs whom Molière ridiculed in his comedy *Le malade imaginaire*;
2) Until 1974, homosexuality figured in the list of mental diseases published by American Psychiatric Association, even though it is just a rather uncommon sexual preference;
3) The cancer attributed to the use of cell phones is impossible because the energy of radio waves is about one-millionth of that of an electromagnetic wave capable of causing a DNA mutation;
4) There is no evidence for the genetic harm attributed to the ingestion of genetically modified vegetables; and
5) Some pharmaceutical firms have invented hormonal deficiencies and mental sicknesses to fit some of their pills.

3.2 Sign: Not Doing Well

The practice of medicine involves translating a patient's complaint into an objective medical report. The patient says, "Doctor, I feel sick, it hurts here." This is a subjective or first-person report. The physician's task is to examine the patient to transform that report into a third-person report of the form "It is possible that the patient suffers from disease X."

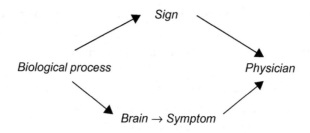

Fig. 3.1. Medical indicators: objective or somatic, and subjective (somatic signals refracted by the feeling and thinking brain).

Thus, whereas the patient lists symptoms (what she feels), her physician looks for the corresponding objective indicators, also called *signs, biomarkers,* and *surrogates.* In other words, patients feel sicknesses, whereas physicians treat diseases, and leave the study and treatment of refractory symptoms, such as chronic pain, to specialists. (See Figure 3.1.)

To repeat: we have assumed that physicians distinguish what their patients tell them (symptoms) from objective signs or biomarkers of what is really going on. This distinction is basically a philosophical one. Indeed, it presupposes *medical realism*, or the assumption that there are diseased people out there. A medical idealist, by contrast, would confuse the two kinds of report. For example, a Kantian — for whom there are only appearances — would claim that a sickness is what the patient feels, so that he would not undertake a detailed examination of the patient, nor order laboratory tests. A follower of Husserl's phenomenology, who is expected to "put the external world in parentheses," will examine his own consciousness rather than the patient before him. A hermeneutician, for whom there are only symbols, would identify the disease with its intuitive diagnosis, without using biomarkers. And a social constructivist would claim that both patient and physician are victims of the latest medical fashion, or even of a dark political conspiracy, so that he would prescribe inaction — even in the case of an epidemic. Only a medical realist will face the problem with due seriousness, even though he won't reject the possibility that his patient suffers from a delusion.

Let us examine more closely the difference between the symptoms one feels and what one really "has." To begin with, the symptoms–signs correspondence is not one-to-one, for there are asymptomatic disorders. For example, one may feel feverish even while having a normal body temperature; hypertension is rightly called "the silent killer" because it has no obvious symptoms; ascariasis, or infection with roundworms, is asymptomatic too; likewise, cancer does not hurt at the beginning, which is why it is usually diagnosed too late; Alzheimer's disease may begin 25 years before any clinical symptoms appear; and the amputee may really feel intense pain in the non-existing or "phantom" limb, for it has remained "represented" on the cerebral cortex, which is subjected to stimuli from other regions of the brain. (See Table 3.1.)

The noted absence of a one-to-one correspondence between symptoms and signs (or biomarkers) is one of the reasons that medical diagnosis can be just as difficult as guessing intention from overt behavior. Another reason is that there are imperceptible biomarkers, like the prostate-specific antigen (PSA), an ambiguous and therefore unreliable prostate cancer indicator.

Imprecision is one of the unfortunate traits of both biomarkers and social indicators, and it is due to their empirical status; they are not backed up by exact and well-confirmed theories. By contrast, these theories explain how the physical and chemical indicators work. For example, they explain why the oscillation period of a simple pendulum is a reliable indicator of the strength of gravity at a place on Earth: because gravity pulls the displaced pendulum back.

It often happens that the law statement that backs up an indicator or marker is true only to a first approximation. For instance, magnetic resonance

Table 3.1. Diseases and corresponding symptoms and signs.

Disease	Symptom	Sign
Diabetes mellitus	Frequent urination	Sugar excess
Lung tuberculosis	Coughing up blood	Excess of Koch bacilli
Anemia	Fatigue	Hemoglobin deficiency
Alzheimer's disease	Cognitive deficits	Aβ accumulation
Hypertension	—	High blood pressure
Ascariasis	—	Roundworms in stools

imaging involves the hypothesis that mental activity is the more intense the stronger the blood flow, which is what the instrument measures. But it has recently been found that an increase in blood flow is not always accompanied by an increase in nervous activity. What is to be done? Clearly, the correlation between blood flow and nervous activity has to be better studied, until a truer law (invariant relation) between the two variables is found. Something like this was done when the first thermometers were recalibrated on the strength of the relation between the temperature and the height of the mercury column; the linear relation was complicated by the addition of a quadratic term. This case illustrates a general pattern: that of the advancement of knowledge through *successive approximations*, along which both the degree of truth and complexity increase.

In conclusion, the best scientific indicators or markers are *well founded* (by contrast with Rorschach's inkblots), as well as both *fallible* and *corrigible* — in contradistinction to those of traditional Asian medicine. This combination of *fallibilism* with *meliorism* is distinctive of *scientific realism*, by contrast to both naïve realism and aprioristic dogmatism.

When the biomarkers themselves are imperceptible, one needs *metaindicators*, or markers of markers, as suggested by the following chain or "hierarchy":

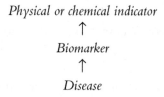

Physical or chemical indicator
↑
Biomarker
↑
Disease

For example, most peptic ulcers are caused by *Helicobacter pylori*, an elusive bacterium. To show the presence of this ulcer biomarker, the patient is asked to drink a liquid containing some radioactive carbon. An hour later, his breath is analyzed. If the said bacteria are there, the patient's breath will contain radioactive carbon dioxide, detectable by means of a Geiger counter. (Incidentally, breath and salivary analyses may soon supplement "blood work" as diagnostic tools.)

Sometimes one or two biomarkers are privileged at the expense of all others, to the point of being regarded as surrogates of a disease. For example, recent research has found that many physicians focused on only two diabetes biomarkers, sugar and insulin, without noticing that their patients were getting blind — like the French joke "he died cured." This mistake has been called "the idolatry of the surrogate" (Yudkin *et al.* 2011).

Seen from afar, the surrogate crisis is not catastrophic, because it emerges as the composition of two common and easily detectable errors. One of them is to take as reliable a biomarker that has not passed all the tests. The other error is to overlook the main point, namely to know whether the patient is getting better. The first error can be corrected with more pharmacological and clinical research. And the second error can be corrected by a more thorough examination and interrogation.

Another problem is the tendency to multiply unnecessarily the number of diseases, as has been common in biological systematics, where new species were invented while only new varieties within a species sufficed. How many diseases are there? Apparently, nobody knows. This ignorance is partly due to the fact that the question has not been well posed. Indeed, the *fundamentum divisionis* has not been explicitly stated: it has not been said whether diseases should be grouped by organ, function, contagiousness, seriousness, etc. Nor are we told whether the groups in question are species, genera, families, or orders of medical disorders.

For example, there are dozens of cardiovascular, gastrointestinal, hepatic, mental, etc. diseases. Hence, whoever counts 20 different diseases — as Cecil's standard textbook (Andreoli *et al.* 2010) does — will be just as right as someone who counts 200, 2,000, or 20,000. It all depends on the predicates one chooses and on their combination.

For example, the class "pulmonary tuberculosis" is formed by conjoining the predicates "tuberculosis" (medical genus) and "pulmonary" (anatomical genus). In turn, that compound predicate can be united with the predicate "disease" (a medical family), resulting in the stupendous compound word occurring in a work of Robert Koch's: *Wundinfektionskrankheiten*.

In any event, there is tacit consent that the International Classification of Diseases, which the WHO publishes periodically, will never be completed. This is because some diseases, like hypertension and autism, turn out to be whole collections ("spectra") of disorders; because new mutations will give rise to new ("emergent") diseases; and because some medical advances will discover previously unknown (but existing) diseases. For example, in recent years, several infectious diseases (like Lyme disease, Ebola, and SARS) have emerged — or perhaps they have been only newly diagnosed; and others (like whooping cough and tuberculosis) have reappeared.

Methodological caution: usually medics, especially psychiatrists, speak of *classifying* diseases, while what they have actually in mind is *categorizing* them. We must define or characterize diseases before attempting to order or class them. Physicians do this every time they play the "20 questions" game in order to reach a diagnosis: severe/minor, acute/chronic, localized/systemic, bacterial/viral, congenital/acquired, communicable/noncommunicable, etc.

Whereas categorizing is grouping *individuals* into taxa, classifying is grouping *species* into genera, genera into families, and so on, as shown in Figure 3.2 in the particular case of five diseases.

There are localized disorders, such as the renal and hepatic ones, whereas others, like the cardiovascular and mental diseases, as well as diabetes, obesity, alcoholism, AIDS, and the hematological diseases, affect the whole body, whence they are called *systemic*. Every subsystem of the body has its specific functions, hence its peculiar disorders, in addition to those that it may share with other organs. For example, only the heart can suffer from arrhythmia, whereas dyspepsia "belongs" to the digestive tract, and depression to the brain. But of course specificity does not imply immutability; the immune system "learns" to resist antigens, the brain reorganizes itself as it learns, and medicine repairs dysfunctions by various means, from bed rest to open-heart surgery, and from compresses to pills.

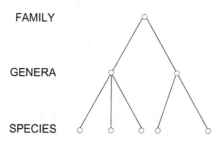

Fig. 3.2. Systematics of five diseases.

Nor does specificity imply the mutual independence of organs; in fact, they are interdependent. In particular, the various "areas" of the brain interact with one another. Such interdependence contradicts the modularity (or Swiss Army knife) conjecture invented by the phrenologists, recently refloated by the philosopher Jerry Fodor, and embraced by the self-styled evolutionary psychologists. This radical version of localizationism is sheer phrenology, since the modules in question are thought of as being inborn, unchanging, and mutually independent.

The modularity hypothesis not only lacks empirical evidence, but is also inconsistent with the finding that the cerebral cortex is connected with the limbic system. In functional terms, cognition and emotion, though distinct, interact with each other, as Damasio (1994) has tirelessly remarked. The prevailing view is that the organs of mental functions are *plastic networks*, rather than hyperspecialized, unchangeable, and mutually independent modules (Fuster 2006).

In other words, the localization of mental functions comes together with their coordination. There would be nothing to coordinate if there were no specialization. A classical example is Geschwind's disconnection syndrome: if the speech "center" (Broca's) is cut off from the speech comprehension "center" (Wernicke's), the patient becomes totally aphasic — he can neither speak nor understand speech.

In modern medicine, all the mental diseases, from inoffensive nervous tics to devastating schizophrenia, are being studied and treated as brain diseases. This was also the Hippocratic and traditional Chinese conception. Until recently, the traditional Chinese doctors, who rejected mind/body dualism, treated mental diseases with acupuncture — without however checking whether or not it worked. Moral: a materialist philosophy does not help medicine unless it inspires biomedical research.

By contrast, shamanism and psychoanalysis regard mental diseases as disorders of the immaterial soul. And psychiatry continues to be separate from neurology even though both deal with dysfunctions of the nervous system (White *et al.* 2012). And the anti-psychiatry movement led by Thomas Szasz, Ronald D. Laing, Michel Foucault, and others denied the existence of mental diseases and claimed that the insane are social non-conformists, that the asylums are tools of political oppression, and that from the start of the nineteenth century, the historical trend has been to institutionalize people in growing numbers. But this is a historical travesty; the asylums have never contained more than 1% of the population, the mentally ill tend to avoid public life, and most of the psychiatric hospitals were closed around 1960, when the first effective antipsychotic drugs reached the market (Shorter 1997). The favorite repression tool of the authoritarian regimes is the jail, not the asylum. The medicalization of politics is as absurd and harmful to public health as the politicization of medicine.

Naturally, in both cases — those of spiritualist psychiatry and anti-psychiatry — the rejection of the hypothesis that the mental is neural has the same practical result: the mental patients do not get the care they need. And this is a serious social problem, in view of the fact that 19.7% of the American population have had some mental illness in 2011 (National Survey on Drug Use and Health, 5 April 2012).

However, criticizing the pseudosciences of the mind does not imply claiming that scientific psychiatry has solved the problem. Everyone agrees that it is the most backward branch of medicine. After all, until recently its progress was held back by a dualist philosophy of mind, and it has advanced only thanks to progress in neuroscience and pharmacology. These advances vindicate the hypothesis that Philippe Pinel proposed shortly after the French Revolution, namely that all mental sicknesses are brain disorders. The same hypothesis led him to introduce his progressive reforms in the treatment of mental patients.

Finally, let us recall stress, whose discovery took the medical community by surprise when Hans Selye's famous book appeared in 1950. Stress is a systemic disorder and, although it neither hurts nor exhibits obvious symptoms, it enlarges some internal organs, alters their functions, and affects farm animals as much as subaltern employees. For example, hens locked up in batteries lay fewer eggs than free-ranging ones. The massive Whitehall Studies (Marmot et al. 1978; Wilkinson 1992) showed that stress affects particularly the low-ranking public servants, who do everything by obligation and live in fear of their superiors (Wilkinson & Pickett 2009). Moreover, chronic stress affects the genome. Indeed, it shortens telomeres (the ends of chromosomes), which in turn has systemic effects such as diabetes and cardiovascular disease (Blackburn & Epel 2012). In sum, medics and psychologists must take note of psychoneuroimmunology (e.g., Kemeny 2009).

Along the same top-down line, Michael Meaney and coworkers (Zhang & Meaney 2010), working with rats, showed that maternal care alters both gene expression and neural function. This finding is only the latest of the pile of facts, uncovered by epigenetics, that confute the nativism of Plato, Lorenz, Chomsky, Dawkins, Pinker, the self-styled evolutionary psychologists, and the "libertarian" ideologues who lead the campaign against public education and universal health care coverage.

At the time of this writing, there is some noise about two alleged personality types: warriors and worriers — with a strong hint of a genetic root. A bit of history should help show that, if the said difference does exist, it has social as well as biological roots. Think, for example, of an Alsatian Frenchman in 1871, turned overnight into a German speaker, taxpayer, pupil, or army recruit just because his country was defeated by the Prussian Army — only to regain his earlier nationality half a century later because of a reversal of political fortunes. Circumstances beyond his control forced him to switch almost overnight from one mood to the other, and then back, though presumably he spent most of his life neither fighting nor brooding. Genes are everywhere in life, but they are not everything in life (see Lewontin & Levins 2007). However, let us go back to medical issues.

Stress is perhaps the most interesting disease for philosophers of mind and social philosophers, because it crosses all the levels of organization, except that of artifacts. In fact, stress is a *psycho-neuro-endocrino-immuno-social* disease, so that its study calls for the convergence of five disciplines. This is one more falsifier of two popular doctrines: nativism and hermeneutics. Nativism is of course the opinion that we are fully products of our biological inheritance: that the environment and learning can at most fine-tune what we bring with us at birth. This thesis has been refuted by the success of maternal care, schooling, and epigenetics — the latest and booming phase of genetics.

A central thesis of hermeneutics is that there is a chasm between culture and nature, hence also between the cultural (or social) and the natural sciences. Of course these disciplines are different, but they overlap partially, and the occurrence of *biosocial facts*, from medical assistance to murder, necessitates the cultivation of *biosociological disciplines*, such as psychology, demography, epidemiology, and social medicine.

The biosociological approach may yield unexpected results — for example, that slavery made the fortune of dentists. How so? Because the West Indies slaves worked the sugarcane plantations, which fed the lucrative British sweets industry. This in turn had two effects: it helped finance the Industrial Revolution, and it increased dramatically the number of people with cavities, from less than 10% to between 50% and 90% of the population in Europe and the USA (Gibbons 2012). In turn, the increase in tooth decay bolstered the dentistry profession, which was a boon to both dentistry faculties and the manufacturers of dental equipment.

Neither a purely biological nor a purely socioeconomic approach could have found out this unexpected relation between slavery, sugar addiction, and massive tooth decay. And yet, the influential "interpretive" (or *Verstehen*) school in the philosophy of social science prohibits crossing the natural–cultural border. This school has not distorted the history of medicine, largely thanks to the pioneering work of Henry Sigerist and his successors in the social history of medicine. Nowadays, few doubt "the incontrovertibly social nature of medicine," as Jones, Podolsky, and Greene (2012) wrote in their overview of the changes in diseases and in medicine over the past two centuries.

3.3 Health and Sickness: Things or Processes?

The most primitive conception of disease is that it is an annoying thing, like a leech, which can be carried, dropped, or transferred. Thus, the Aztecs believed that everyone is born with the same lifespan of 52 years, which could be increased by stealing a piece of someone else's lifespan, whence oldsters were looked upon with suspicion and fear (Mata Pinzón 2009). This view is often mistakenly called "ontological." This is a misnomer, because there are dynamical or processual ontologies, from Heraclitus to Hegel to Whitehead.

The view of sickness as a thing is entrenched in ordinary language. In fact, we often say "I have a cold" as if we were wearing a piece of clothing. But this is only an example of the thesis that ordinary language is coarse and full of conceptual fossils. It also exhibits the magico–religious idea of a disease as a thing received as punishment or revenge, and that can be unloaded onto others. Thus, until not so long ago, some sick people pretended to place their disease in an attractive little box that they dropped on a sidewalk. Whoever picked it up was saddled with the disease.

But of course, health and sickness, though changeable, are not things that may be worn or changed like shirts. As Virchow and Bernard pointed out, diseases are *states* or *conditions* of things of a very special kind, namely living systems. This is how the WHO defined health in 1946: "Health is a state of complete physical, mental and social well-being and not merely the absence of disease or infirmity."

Now, if Health = Well-being, then Sickness = Feeling unwell. Note that well-being and discomfort are subjective: an individual may feel well even while being hypertensive or cancerous; or she may feel ill even while being healthy — as is often the case with hypochondriacs. Hence, as several experts have pointed out, the definition in question is imperfect.

Note that the WHO picks the health concept out of the blue rather than from a definite context, as required by a systemic approach to the problem. Now, the proper context of the dual concepts of health and disease is the whole of biology, for they are properties of organisms rather than autonomous things. Indeed what is common to all diseases is that they threaten life.

This simple idea presupposes the complex idea of life, which is no less than the core of biology, and therefore the central problem of the philosophy of biology (see Mahner & Bunge 1997). This is exactly how the dual ideas of health and disease are handled by the present author (Bunge 1979: 86–88). Suppose we know which the defining or essential traits — properties and mechanisms (functions) — of an organism are, such as containing lipids and nucleic acids, feeding, metabolizing, and synthesizing proteins. Then we propose the following definitions (op. cit.: 86):

healthy organism = one that discharges all those essential (vital) functions and

disease = disruption of one or more such functions.

Regardless of the flaws in the WHO's definition of 'health,' what matters most is that it conceives correctly of disease as a *state* and not as an entity or thing. (The word 'condition' is often used as a synonym of 'state.') No disease can be acquired or lost, discarded or transferred as if it were a thing detachable from the organisms that suffer it. For this reason, we should say "I am sick" instead of "I have a sickness" or "I caught a disease."

This difference is not only linguistic but also logical. Indeed, "I have a cancer" has the form "Hab," where H = have, a = me, and b = cancer. By contrast, the logical form of "a is cancerous" is "Ca." In the preceding formulas, the letters H and C designate *predicates*, whereas a and b stand for *individuals*. While the predicate C is *unary* or one-placed, H is *binary* or two-placed; whereas C applies to single individuals, H applies to pairs of individuals. There are also ternary predicates, such as "to treat," in "a treats b with c" and others of a higher order. The most common relations, such as "greater than" and "less widespread than," are binary (two-placed) predicates or *relations*. The mathematical *functions* of the form "$y = f(x)$" constitute a particular case of a relation: that where every value of the independent variable x is paired to a single value of the dependent variable y.

True, we often speak of the contagion or transmission of diseases, but as a matter of fact what gets transmitted in the case of an infectious disease is not the disorder but the bacteria or viruses that cause it. And in the case of unhealthy behaviors, there is more or less deliberate imitation rather than transmission proper.

What is a state? A state of a concrete thing at a given time is the list of its properties at that instant. Example: the list of vital signs of a person when examined by a physician. Now, all concrete things, from photons to cells to humans to social groups, have a number of properties or traits. Think of the long list of properties of an adult individual: age, weight, height, vital signs, occupation, social position, etc.

In exceptional cases, one is interested in a single salient property or sign of the thing under study, to the point that it may suffice for medical diagnosis — though of course not for understanding the underlying mechanism. For example, in humans, anemia is defined as the state of a person whose concentration of red blood cells is lower than $7\,g/dL$. This parameter suffices for diagnosing anemia, though of course not for understanding or curing it since, although it is much deeper than the corresponding syndrome (paleness and fatigue), it says nothing about the possible causes of the deficiency in question.

The main causes of anemia are internal, such as intestinal hemorrhage and menstruation. It has been known since ancient times that iron "fights" anemia. But the cause of this was found out only in 1959, when Max Perutz revealed the molecular structure of the hemoglobin molecule.

It turned out that there is an iron atom at the center of the heme molecule — which, together with the globulin molecule, comprise the hemoglobin molecule — and each iron atom can bind with up to four oxygen atoms. Hence, when there is iron deficiency, hemoglobin synthesis slows down, as a consequence of which oxygen transport is decreased — a deficiency that is translated into anemia, which in turn appears (is manifested) as paleness and extreme fatigue. And, as blood is lost, the body produces more hemoglobin, until the iron supply becomes insufficient. The same mechanism also explains the therapeutic effectiveness of the drugs containing iron or iron compounds, as well as the inefficiency of the rest.

None of this would be known if the biomedical researchers had listened to the warnings of the philosophers who, from Hume and Kant to their positivist successors, were so bent on discrediting religion that they banned all the theories that go beyond appearances. Even though it has the virtues of clarity and demanding empirical evidence, this stance, *phenomenalism*, was an obstacle to the advancement of knowledge.

Galileo's trial was basically that of realism, since the defendant had adopted the realism inherent in heliocentric astronomy against the phenomenalism and conventionalism of the defenders of the geocentric model (Duhem 1908). Paradoxically, none of the secular empiricists and phenomenalists of the next three centuries, from Hume and Kant to the members of the Vienna Circle and the defenders of the Copenhagen interpretation of quantum mechanics, realized that they had adopted the philosophy of Galileo's judges.

Scientists overcame phenomenalism when they constructed and confirmed field physics, microphysics, atomic chemistry, genetics, and cosmology, and when physicians sought out the objective if imperceptible processes behind symptoms. And medics tacitly discarded phenomenalism when they ceased to regard the color, smell, and taste of urine as critical biomarkers, and shifted their gaze to such imperceptibles as red blood cell count, blood pressure, and metabolic rate.

And yet, speculation about *qualia*, or felt qualities, such as colors, smells, and pains, is at the center of contemporary metaphysics and philosophy of mind (see Block *et al.* 2002). The reason is that physics cannot explain qualia or phenomena, which constitute a neat confutation of physicalism.

But, since qualia occur in brains, they are material processes that cognitive neuroscience is equipped to account for. Hence, the existence of qualia refutes physicalism, the most primitive kind of materialism, but it confirms systemic and emergent materialism.

This episode is reminiscent of the mechanism/vitalism dilemma at the center of the philosophy of biology in the nineteenth century; it too was overcome by systemic emergentism, which admits, indeed stresses, the supraphysical properties of organisms (see Mahner & Bunge 1997).

How can diseases be represented mathematically? A good start is to think of a *state vector* — the list of the salient properties of a diseased body. In the simplest case, that of deficiencies and excesses of a biological parameter, the vector contracts to a line segment, as shown in Figure 3.3.

In the vast majority of cases, more than one biomarker is required to represent a state of health or of sickness. Correspondingly, a box in a Cartesian space of several dimensions will be required, every side of which represents a biological parameter (Bunge 1979; Thurler *et al.* 2003). Think of the four-dimensional abstract space generated by the four standard vital signs: pulse rate, temperature, respiration rate, and blood pressure. (The last is actually a couple of numbers.) This may be called the *vital state space*. Every point of it represents schematically a state of health — good, poor, or medium.

A state space is an abstract space unrelated to the three-dimensional physical space, and it is not a metric space, so that there is no distance proper between health states. Every state of health or of sickness of an organism will correspond to a point inside a box. This box will have as many dimensions as the number of properties being considered, and every side of it will coincide with the interval within which the organism is healthy or sick.

The course of a disease will be represented by a continuous curve joining a health-point to a disease-point in the state space. The death states will be confined within a box around the origin of the state space, which is the

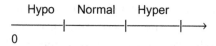

Fig. 3.3. One-dimensional state space: a single biomarker, such as sugar concentration in blood: hypoglycemia–normal–hyperglycemia.

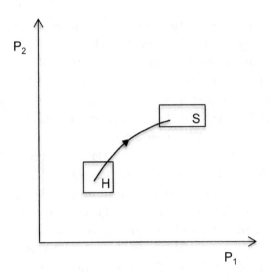

Fig. 3.4. Representation of the course of a disease in a state space with coordinates P_1 and P_2. The boxes H and S represent sets of healthy and sick states, respectively (redrawn from Thurler *et al*. 2003).

intersection of its axes. So, the recipe for staying alive is simple: dwell outside this particular box. (See Figure 3.4.)

Thus, the concept of a state space allows one to analyze the notion of disease as a *process* or *sequence of states*, also called *course of a disease* rather than as a single state. Although this process is continuous, it has been known since antiquity that it may be divided into stages. A tragic example is that of untreated syphilis. Another is the family of the so-called dynamical diseases, such as malaria and epilepsy, characterized by periodicity and caused by abnormalities in the underlying control mechanisms (Mackey & Glass 1977).

The course of a viral disease may be followed quantitatively by measuring the viral load and the rates of production and loss of virions, which in the case of AIDS is about 10^{10} per day. The variation of these rates and the viral load in the course of a disease over a decade may be translated into a system of linear differential equations that not only models the HIV dynamics, but also guides the experimental investigation of it, if only because it identifies the variables that must be measured (Perelson 2002).

When no measurable biomarkers are available, physicians resort to qualitative descriptions of disabilities. For example, in patients with cardiac disorders, the intensity of the disability is equated with their functional capacity, or ability to perform everyday activities. Thus, four kinds or degrees of disability result: intact, slightly compromised, moderately compromised, and severely compromised capacity. In turn, the functional status is evaluated by symptoms such as fatigue, dyspnea, and palpitations, both at rest and when walking on a treadmill. And some of these symptoms, in particular fatigue, have measurable signs. Thus, modern medicine, just like physics, attempts to put into practice Galileo's slogan: *Measure everything measurable.*

The genetic diseases, like gigantism and progeria, might seem to escape the quantitative conception of the normal and the pathological. Not so, because every disorder with a genetic origin is reducible to the insufficient or excessive expression of a gene or gene complex. For example, carcinogens act by combining with DNA molecules, thus inhibiting some of their functions, such as slowing down their mitotic rate, which translates into cell proliferation, whence the therapeutic promise of apoptosis to control cancer growth. Note the mention of a genetic *mechanism*. This is rare in the field of genetic associations, which abounds in papers hastily asserting the existence of amazing gene–disease correlations that are seldom replicated (Moonesinghe *et al.* 2007).

What about mental diseases? When conceived of as brain disorders, they fall in principle within the reach of the state-space approach. In fact, one might use the concentrations of the relevant neurotransmitters and the firing rates of key neural networks among other parameters (Bunge 1977b). Such a research project is inconceivable in either a spiritualist or a dualist perspective, where the mental is detachable from the material. However, we must admit that neuroscience, psychology, and psychiatry have yet to identify and measure all the coordinates needed to place the normal and abnormal regions in a state space for a human brain. A start might be made by doing this for a part of a brain of a simpler organism, yet one capable of having mental experiences, such as perceiving and feeling pain.

To make a speculative leap into the future: medicine could be viewed as the discipline that seeks to identify the state spaces for all major diseases, so as to improve the position of individuals in them. And social medicine would seek to maintain whole populations within the health boxes inside such abstract spaces. To attain this goal, it is incumbent on statesmen and concerned citizens to frame and put into practice preventive social policies regarding immunization, sanitation, environmental contamination, city planning, housing, jobs, education, health care, and the control of guns and toxic products such as alcohol and tobacco. We will return to this subject in Chapter 8.

Clearly, the preceding is an oversimplified description of the multifarious and enormous task that the biomedical researchers and health care workers perform. In this description, there are no traces of the pain, anguish, and stress that accompany the sickness and caregiving experiences. But this is the price we must pay if we wish to gain general, clear, and adequate concepts of health and its dual, namely sickness. In general, abstraction facilitates generalization. And once some general hypotheses (or else rules) have been obtained, they may be applied to many particular cases.

Those unwilling to pay this price risk getting lost in the confusion of daily medical assistance; instead of guiding their patients, the physicians will be dragged by them. This is what happened to Canguilhem (1966) and his followers, who focused on the "suffering subjective body" — they never went beyond homespun psychology.

(Moreover, Canguilhem fell into the linguistic trap: *souffrant*, literally *in pain*, is the French equivalent of *sick*. Those who, like Canguilhem and Wittgenstein, stick to ordinary language, won't seek to unveil the mechanism(s) underlying the disease process, hence won't be able to alter it. *Res, non verba!*)

Last, but not least, let us remember that, by definition, every serious disease comes with "complications" or comorbidities. For instance, hypertension affects not only the cardiovascular system but also the kidneys, brain, and eyes. Another clear example is any serious vision impairment; e.g., people with cataracts tend to trip and suffer hip fractures more often than those with normal vision. That diseases come in clusters, and consequently must be treated as such rather than one by one, will not surprise the systemist philosopher: recall Section 2.3.

Coda

Although the job of physicians has always been that of treating the sick, there is no consensus on what diseases are. Lay people emphasize symptoms, what one feels, whereas the modern physicians seek objective signs.

But neither of them tells us what a disease itself is, regardless of its manifestations. The ancient Egyptians believed that each disease was caused by a given god. The Aztecs knew that the gods have better things to do, and believed that diseases are caused by sorcerers. And the constructivist-relativists claim that diseases are social constructions, perhaps fabrications of evil pharmaceutical firms, or even political conspiracies. Only naturalists believe that diseases are natural processes, usually with deep but in principle controllable underlying mechanisms. Modern physicians take this philosophical assumption for granted although they do not call it 'philosophical.'

Obviously, the treatment of a medical disorder will depend on the nature to which it is attributed. Those who believe that diseases result from curses of sorcerers or punishment by supernatural beings will try to bribe them or to appease them with sacrifices — human if necessary, as the Incas believed. If diseases are attributed to "bad thoughts" or "complexes," confession and penance (or a fine) will be indicated. Only those who regard diseases as somatic dysfunctions will seek treatment through physical, chemical, biological, or social interventions. And only those who adopt the scientific method will demand empirical tests, such as clinical trials. The others will remain content with testimonials.

The medics who adopt a secular and naturalistic conception of diseases will describe or even explain them, and if they are also science-oriented, they will only use well-tested therapies. Some physicians in ancient Egypt and ancient Greece described correctly the symptoms of several diseases, but they could explain very few of them because of a lack of the requisite biomedical knowledge, which started to emerge only in the mid-sixteenth century.

Aristotle was a keen marine biologist, but he was not interested in the human body, which was studied by some of his disciples, in particular Theophrastus. And nearly two millennia later, Descartes described the human optical nerve in physical terms, but could not explain vision because this phenomenon occurs in the brain, then uncharted territory, and anyhow he believed that the mental is immaterial. Even today, most philosophers of mind ignore the neurosciences, even if they call themselves materialists. In fact, they are functionalists, and as a consequence they are of no help to psychiatry.

Despite his limitations, Aristotle exerted on the whole a beneficial influence on medicine because of his insistence that new knowledge can come only from research rather than from reading old books — advice that, alas, most of his followers did not heed. And, in conceiving of the body as a machine, Descartes paved the way to biophysics and biochemistry. It is possible that, as has often been said, this view made the dissection of human corpses more acceptable; what is sure is that it facilitated the ill treatment of laboratory animals.

A start for a deep understanding of disease mechanisms came only with the emergence of cellular biology, biochemistry, pharmacology, and bacteriology in the nineteenth century. These advances, in turn, led to inventing and trying out radical therapies, that is, treatments that attack the sources of sicknesses rather than their symptoms. However, before dealing with therapies we must study diagnosis and medicaments, as well as their evaluation.

Chapter 4

DIAGNOSIS

4.1 Diagnostic Reasoning

Laymen tend to diagnose medical problems by analogy and on the strength of anecdotes and testimonials; moreover, they do not keep count of their hits, much less of their misses. Doctors too use analogies and exemplary cases, but their casuistry is professional; they examine their patients before diagnosing them and prescribing treatments. And they do both things on the strength of long and usually demanding studies. (By contrast, typically, the quack has no serious medical background, and learns his trade in a few weeks.) In some cases, the medical problem is in clear view: runny nose, flesh wound, skin ulcer, trauma, deformity, paralysis, obesity, and so on. But many patients "seen" by physicians suffer internal disorders, from hypertension to depression, that call for more-or-less deep studies. And that's where philosophy raises its head.

Most of the problems tackled by internal medicine are hard for several reasons. First, most patients do not know what is wrong with them except for the symptoms they feel. Second, self-diagnoses by lay people are often incorrect; for example, one may blame the wrong tooth for a toothache. Third, many symptoms are ambiguous. And fourth, symptoms are manifestations of processes that are often imperceptible. For example, until around 1900, syphilis was regarded as a skin disease, and hence was treated by dermatologists, just because its early symptoms are skin ulcers. Psychiatry is the only branch of medicine where symptomatic diagnosis still prevails — a clear sign of its backwardness.

However, the main reason for the inherent difficulty of correct diagnoses is that diagnosis is a typically *inverse problem*, that is, one from going back from mouth to source, from effect to cause, from syndrome to mechanism, from present to past, or from conclusion to premises. And, as will be seen below, inverse problems are far tougher than their direct duals, because they have multiple solutions or none. On top of being an inverse problem, diagnosis is exposed to the traps of spontaneous and quick reasoning. Perhaps the most common of these traps is the halo effect — the "anchoring" to first impressions, data, or guesses (Kahneman 2011). But another two fallacies are nearly as frequent as the former: the leap from statistical correlation to causation, and *post hoc, ergo propter hoc.*

Let us start at the beginning: the examination of a patient who has just arrived at a medical clinic. The doctor does not attempt to observe *all* the traits of the patient, for this would be impossible; instead, he confines himself to the *key variables*, such as posture and blood pressure, as well as to the *suspected variables*, those suggested by the story he has just heard, as well as by the patient's clinical history. Variables of both kinds occur in clinical conjectures of two types: the *heuristic* ones, which evaluate the relevant variables, and the *substantive* ones, which point to the possible disorder.

For example, if the patient is obese, the clinician may suspect sugar excess, which in turn is a biomarker of diabetes mellitus. However, this is only one of the diseases that stalk the obese. There are further possibilities, from injured knees caused by overweight to a cognitive deficiency caused by the insulin excess that accompanies the digestion of excessive food. (In fact, the brain contains hormones that interfere with neurotransmitters, and others, such as dopamine, which double as neurotransmitters.)

That is, from the moment he meets his patient, the physician frames rapidly, one after another, several educated guesses (hypotheses) about the kind of disease and its possible causes (Groopman 2008). But, far from adopting any of them right away, the good (and unhurried) physician seeks *evidence* relevant to the more plausible conjectures he has formulated. And if the examination he has just concluded does not reduce significantly his uncertainty, he orders one or more tests, such as blood work.

For instance, if the patient is a pregnant woman with a history of spontaneous miscarriages, her physician may prescribe an amniocentesis to look for developmental abnormalities of the fetus. Such exploration will be censored by those who oppose human interference in the implementation of divine designs. The same should apply to all the other invasive interventions, from immunization to blood transfusion to appendectomy to insertion of catheters to organ transplant. Obviously, these operations raise serious practical, moral, and theological issues.

One of the practical problems is raised by the abuse of invasive examinations, such as endoscopies, biopsies, and X-rays. For instance, we now know that not every swollen ankle calls for an X-ray; that it is not necessary to conduct colonoscopies more than every five years; and that consecutive prostate biopsies are counterindicated unless there are significant clinical signs of gland enlargement.

In short, in the prosperous countries, we suffer from overdiagnosis (Welch *et al.* 2011). For example, three decades of screening mammography on breast cancer incidence in the USA have shown that "the benefit of mortality reduction is probably smaller, and the harm of overdiagnosis probably larger, than has been previously recognized" (Bleyer & Welch 2012). This might be the time for setting up a scientific task force to find out the lowest carcinogenic X-ray dose.

An excess of clinical data may be as harmful to medicine as a severe data scarcity, if only because a person's mind cannot juggle more than a handful of variables at a time. And the hope that a computer may take over when the number of variables is large is illusory, because computers cannot generate new ideas; they are only good at processing extant ideas with clever programs.

The philosopher will note that medical practice satisfies neither the dogmatic apriorist who claims to know without observing nor the empiricist who recommends seeking data in the dark. The good physician combines hypotheses with data, the way Claude Bernard (1865) recommended; he is what may be called a *ratioempiricist* — a hybrid of Hercule Poirot and Sherlock Holmes. (Incidentally, Kant and the logical empiricists of the 1930s attempted to synthesize rationalism with empiricism, but their valiant attempts failed due to their attachment to phenomenalism, or the cult of appearances. Ratioempiricism is fruitful only jointly with realism.)

The data available to an up-to-date physician are so many and so varied, that to understand them, much more knowledge is needed than the one that the best nineteenth-century physician could muster. It suffices to look at the form of a "blood work," which includes biomarkers unknown until a few decades ago. The doctor will not ask that all of them be measured, but only those that are suspect in light of the office examination, the clinical history, and the relevant statistical data for populations of individuals of similar characteristics. Perhaps he tacitly uses Pareto's 80–20 rule of thumb: that 80% of facts can be explained by 20% of variables.

Let us peep at the way a contemporary physician reasons when intent on diagnosing a medical disorder. His starting point is the tacit hypothesis that every disease manifests itself as a bundle of signs or indicators, only some of which (the symptoms) the patient can feel, and some of which he will forget or even be reluctant to reveal (recall Section 3.1). It is tempting, though fallacious, to leap from symptom to disorder, the way shamans and traditional doctors did. This is wrong because different diseases may share nearly the same syndrome, particularly at the initial stages. For example, both the common cold and pulmonary tuberculosis start with slight fever and coughing.

This explains why, when objective biomarkers are unavailable, early diagnoses are often wrong — as is often the case with mental disorders in adolescence, when the brain is awash in hormones, some of which, like dopamine, are neurotransmitters. By contrast, when objective signs are available, a disease can be defined by both *kind* and *intensity*, so that category mistakes — e.g., of depression for schizophrenia — may be avoided, and consequently the correct treatment can be prescribed.

The true relation between a disease D and its objective signs or biomarkers S is not the conditional "If S, then D," but its converse, "If D, then S." Let us emphasize that S stands for a conjunction of objective (and often measurable) signs, not for subjective indicators such as the feelings of satiety, insecurity, or anxiety. In scientific medicine, a hypothesis of this kind is put to the experimental test. When D is the case and S is observed, the formula is said to be confirmed, and falsified if S fails to appear. But of course, such logical validity is medically worthless, because the point of a diagnosis is to identify D from S. We shall address this conundrum below. But first a caution.

If a single sign, such as glycemia, is available, the physician may take either of these approaches: the dogmatic (or hasty), or the skeptical (or prudent). The former consists in identifying disease with some signs (surrogates), pushing the remaining signs aside. The skeptic, by contrast, will frame two or more hypotheses that look plausible in light of his antecedent knowledge — what he had before facing the given problem.

In this case, D will equal the disjunction of several propositions — as many as the diseases accompanied by the same signs. The next step will be to check every one of these conceptual possibilities, until all but one of them have been discarded, so that the diagnosis problem will have been solved — until further notice.

However, let us backtrack. If we assume a hypothesis of the form *If D, then S*, the basic rule of logic, *modus ponens*, allows us to reason as follows: if a given individual b suffers from disease D, then he will exhibit signs S. Now, b does suffer from D. Hence, b exhibits S (in other words: Law & Circumstance $\therefore$ Diagnosis or prognosis). Unfortunately, this argument is as useless for diagnosis as it is logically impeccable. Indeed, what the doctor needs to solve is the *inverse* problem: going from S to D. But logic blocks this road. Hence, the doctor is forced to build a new road, or rather a precarious footpath in the wilderness; he will enrich the initial set S of signs with the results of a new battery of tests. With luck, he will make an educated and inspired guess: what ails b is likely to be D. The physician will accordingly prescribe the standard therapy for D patients, and check whether it works.

If the patient does not improve with the new therapy, the diagnosis will have been falsified, and a new one will have to be guessed and tried. A new hypothesis, involving a different disease D', and possibly a somewhat different set S' of signs, may call for further tests. If the new tests, involving some new biomarkers, succeed, the diagnosis problem will finally have been solved.

Still, even if the correct diagnosis has been found, a fresh problem will emerge: that of adopting or devising the corresponding treatment. If the patient responds positively to it, the hypotheses concerning disease and treatment will have been confirmed. Otherwise, at least one of them will turn out to be false.

Such disease and treatment failures will be annoying but should not be surprising, because no two individuals get sick or react to medication in exactly the same way, as different people have different clinical histories and different immune systems. Consequently, the zigzagging between diagnoses and treatments is bound to be longer and less successful in some cases than in others, as shown by the existence of chronic diseases and fatal outcomes. But all new and interesting medical failures will be recorded and studied to the benefit of future generations, contrary to mistakes in traditional medicines, which are quietly buried or cremated.

What if the disease is so new that doctors cannot diagnose it, much less treat it, as happened in recent times with AIDS, SARS, and Ebola? This is a tragedy for those afflicted by such a disease, but a golden opportunity for biomedical researchers, as they can write research grant proposals bound to receive preferential attention. This is one of the advantages of science: that in this field ignorance spurs action, whereas elsewhere it paralyzes or misdirects it.

Note two salient traits of medical diagnosis: the abundance of hypotheses and frequent occurrence of inverse problems, of the *Signs* → *Disease* type. Indeed, contrary to popular belief, the good doctor is not a good empiricist; he does not stick by what he sees, smells, or touches, nor does he proceed with the assurance of the healer, but is uncertain much of the time, and frames, tries out, and discards hypotheses. Moreover, when framing hypotheses, the doctor makes ample use of his professional knowledge — what he learned at medical school plus what he has read in medical journals and heard at specialized symposia, or while making hospital rounds in the company of more experienced colleagues.

In short, good doctors are neither blind data hunters nor uncritical believers in tradition. Instead, they use the *experimental method*, which may be condensed into the following sequence of steps:

background knowledge–problem–solution candidate (hypothesis, experimental design, or technique)–test of candidate–eventual revision of either solution candidate, checking the procedure, background knowledge, or even problem.

The medic *discovers* facts and *invents* hypotheses and procedures. The fashionable opinion that there is a science of discovery different from hypotheses-driven research has no historical basis. Even chance discoveries result from explorations motivated by hypotheses. As Louis Pasteur famously said, "Chance favors only the prepared mind." I went in search of *A* and did not find it; instead, I found *B*. This is called *serendipity* (see Merton & Barber 2004).

In sum, the good medic guesses all the time. But his guesses are educated, not fantastic; he imagines and tries out *biologically possible*, not merely conceivable, things or processes. Of course, even the most plausible medical hypothesis may turn out to be false. When this happens, alternative hypotheses are tried out until the least false one is found. True, we sometimes delay admitting that we were wrong, particularly if such admission may be used as evidence in a malpractice trial. But this only goes to show that the search for truth involves honesty: no science without conscience.

The preceding explains why there is often room for a second opinion — different physicians may frame different hypotheses to account for the same set of data concerning a difficult case, because they have different brains, sculpted by somewhat different learning experiences and interests. Evidently, different opinions about the same problem may be either mutually exclusive or complementary. This is why it is important that the various doctors who studied the same difficult case get together to discuss it, seeking a consensus, as is often done in teaching hospitals.

Obviously, for such a discussion to be fruitful, it is necessary that all the participants belong to the same medical tradition, as well as to the philosophies according to which reason and evidence trump dogma and intuition. Therefore, the attempts to reconcile scientific medicine with traditional medicine, like those recently sponsored by the World Health Organization, are as pointless as the efforts to reconcile religion with science.

Last, but not least, all diagnostic problems raise inverse problems of the type *Signs* → *Disease*. To solve these we only have solutions to one or more direct problems of the form *Disease* → *Signs*. Regrettably, most logicians and philosophers have ignored the very existence of inverse problems, even though they are the hardest and therefore the more interesting ones.

This holds especially for the believers in the computer model of the mind, because there can be no algorithms for tackling such problems; every one of them calls for new hypotheses. Charles Peirce called *abduction* the resorting to conjecturing when both induction and deduction fail. But he did not make the mistake of regarding abduction as a *method* or regular procedure; he warned that it is nothing but conjecturing. (More on inverse problems in Bunge 2006.)

Every Nobel Prize in science or medicine is expected to reward the finding of a new and important fact pointed to by a hypothesis or due to an original experimental design. That prize is never awarded for more precise measurement results or more precise computations. As Comte de Buffon, the earliest scientific evolutionary scientist, might have said, the Nobel Prize rewards inspiration, not perspiration. In particular, it recompenses the solution of important inverse problems, which are feats of controlled imagination.

Back to the methodology of inverse problems. The procedure described above can be considerably improved if the purely descriptive hypothesis *If D, then S* is combined with conjectures about the possible mechanisms involved in the start and course of disease *D*. Some mechanisms, such as cuts and burns, are perceptible. But most of them, such as infection, internal hemorrhage, artery obstruction, failure of the immune system, and mutation, are imperceptible. Therefore, they have to be conjectured and studied to check whether they have been acting.

How are *mechanismic* (or *mechanistic*) hypotheses framed? This is hard to know. It is easier to know how they are *not* usually born; they do not emerge from induction, that is, by generalization from empirical data, because most mechanisms are imperceptible, and induction starts from empirical data. For example, we know from experience that vaccinations immunize almost completely, but only immunological research can tell us why (namely because a brush with the given disease stimulates the synthesis of antibodies). Nor do mechanismic hypotheses emerge by deduction, since they involve the invention of new concepts, that is, of concepts that do not belong in the antecedent knowledge (Bunge 2012b).

If a mechanismic hypothesis is explicitly formulated, maybe someone will come up with a procedure to put it to the test. For instance, if a patient suffers from persistent coughing, the first hypothesis is laryngitis, which can be checked, if necessary with the help of a laryngoscope. If the larynx proves innocent, the doctor may suspect bronchitis, which can be discovered by simple auscultation with the help of a stethoscope. But if the airways prove to be clear, the lung will be the third suspect, and this will require a sputum analysis and an X-ray. In the vast majority of cases, the cause of the ailment, or necessary and sufficient condition for its occurrence, will finally be found. However, in some cases, the mechanism is very well hidden, as happens when the immune system "fights" a pathogen and delays the appearance of signs and symptoms, so that the "aggressor" remains latent for a long time.

At other times the triggering event is in view, but its link to the symptom is unclear. This is the case of shell shock, or post-traumatic stress disorder (PTSD), attributed to 30.9% of the Vietnam War veterans; the cause is combat with a resilient enemy in an unfriendly territory. What about the similar disorder suffered by non-combatants, particularly children, under bombardment and military occupation? We do not know much about them because they are only "collateral damage," and anyway they cannot benefit from the U.S. Department of Veteran Affairs.

However, PTSD is not well defined, since its symptoms — insomnia, anxiety, and recurrent nightmares — have no clear objective counterparts. Moreover, they are shared by sufferers from other mental disorders, and they can be felt even in the absence of the traumatizing event. In this case, the patient suffers, but the causes are still hidden (Rosen & Lilienfeld 2008). And, because the etiology of PTSD is unknown, no treatment has been found for it. Once again, philosophical advice is indicated: *Primum cognoscere, deinde medicari.*

If the disease mechanism that has been conjectured is biologically plausible, it will be possible to use two laws instead of one: the disease–mechanism, and the mechanism–signs conjectures. In standard symbols: $D \Rightarrow S$ can be analyzed into the conjunction $(D \Rightarrow M)$ & $(M \Rightarrow S)$. For example,

Arthrosis $\Rightarrow$ Rigid joints

may be analyzed into

Arthrosis $\Rightarrow$ Calcium carbonate deposits in joints

and

Calcium carbonate deposits in joints $\Rightarrow$ Rigid joints.

In turn, pain is the symptom corresponding to the objective indicator rigid joints. I propose calling *strong diagnosis* the mechanism-based diagnosis.

Let us finally examine the exceptional case where there is a single biologically plausible mechanism, such as the one of AIDS. This mechanism is so insidious that the famous virologist Peter Duesberg, the first to discover a cancer gene, and the chemist Kary Mullis, who won the Nobel Prize for inventing the polymerase chain reaction, denied the malignity of the new disease as well as the hypothesis that it is caused by the HIV. This denial obstructed AIDS research and led the South African government to delay for years the use of the antiretroviral therapy. This policy resulted in an estimated 330,000 unnecessary deaths, all of them victims of the abuse of both scientific and political authority (Nattrass 2012).

AIDS does not break out suddenly; it develops when the organism is invaded by the HIV and, at the same time, the immune system fails because its reaction cannot keep pace with the virions' reproduction. In short, *AIDS occurs ⟺ HIV invasion & Slow immune reaction*, where ⟺ is interpreted as "if and only if." In other words, HIV infection and immune failure are jointly necessary and sufficient for the full development of AIDS.

Whenever the mechanism M of a disease D is both necessary and sufficient for D, the conditionals ($\Rightarrow$) involved in the previous discussion can be replaced with the corresponding biconditionals ($\Leftrightarrow$). This is how certainty discards the uncertainty that accompanies weak diagnosis. Indeed, the logical form of the diagnostic reasoning is now

$$(D \Leftrightarrow M) \ \& \ (M \Leftrightarrow S) \ \therefore \ (D \Leftrightarrow S).$$

More explicitly,

For all x: $(Dx \Leftrightarrow Mx)$ & *For all x*: $(Mx \Leftrightarrow Sx)$ $\therefore$ *For all x*: $(Dx \Leftrightarrow Sx)$.

The application to a particular individual b is

For all x: $(Dx \Leftrightarrow Sx)$ & Sb $\therefore$ Db.

In other words, precise data about the disease's signs, jointly with some knowledge of its mechanism, allow one to *transform an inverse problem into a direct one*, and an erratic reasoning into a logically valid and certain argument. Moreover, such reasoning can be "mechanized," that is, incorporated into programs fed into the expert systems employed in informatized medical diagnosis. These machines avoid inadvertent biases and save time, hence also lives — provided they are fed sound science.

However, like any technological advancement, the mechanization of reasoning has its dark side — it may lead to adopting the dogma *machina dixit*. To avoid this risk, one has always to remember that the hypotheses involved in automatized reasoning are fallible and therefore subject to correction as research keeps going. (For example, the fact that the symptoms of heart failure are not the same in women as in men was discovered only recently.) Incidentally, contrary to what Karl Popper (1935) taught, science does not advance by refuting conjectures, but by finding new truths, from data to theories, only some of which contradict old ones. Likewise, farms do not prosper by just weeding, since what they sell are edibles, not weeds.

The computer is yet to reach psychopathology, and it won't be helpful before this discipline completes its morphing from protoscience into science. This transformation started in the mid-1950s with the discovery of the first effective psychopharmaceutical drugs — a fact that ruined the psychoanalytic industry everywhere except in Paris, Barcelona, and Buenos Aires. (In the latter there is a quarter officially called Villa Freud.)

Since that pharmacological breakthrough, most psychiatrists learned Alcmaeon's materialist hypothesis, embraced by Hippocrates, that every-thing mental is cerebral. In turn, this hypothesis entails Philippe Pinel's, that all mental disorders are cerebral — as any victim of stroke or concus-sion will agree. (This applies to severe diseases such as deep depression and schizophrenia, not to inappropriate behaviors, such as living tethered to a cell phone. Because they have been learned, these abnormal behav-iors can be unlearned without major neural alterations or the help of psychotropic drugs.)

A materialist philosophy may guide a research project, but it cannot replace it. Half a century ago, when psychotropic drugs replaced psycho-analytic myths, the psychiatric profession gained in pills and in grateful patients, but remained with few ideas. True, cognitive (and affective) neu-roscience supplied some clues, but these did not help inventing correct diagnoses or designing reliable therapies. Psychiatrists still proceed largely by trial and error, and most of their chronic patients, particularly the severely depressed, are nearly as helpless as before. Although doubt is pref-erable to dogma, since the former may spur while the latter paralyzes, in professional practice, one needs a modicum of trust in what one is doing. And nowadays, psychiatrists tend to be rather skeptical about the power of their science.

Scientific psychiatry is still so backward, that it even lacks a good categorization of mental diseases; the standard one is symptomatic, which is as if dermatologists characterized skin diseases by their color alone. Indeed, there are no reliable biomarkers of mental disorders; only behav-ioral and subjective symptoms, such as memory loss, anxiety, and halluci-nation, are used to diagnose them, even when they are suspected to have different underlying mechanisms. Worse, deep depression, paranoia, and schizophrenia share so many symptoms that they are often confused with one another, and consequently treated with roughly the same drugs. Moreover, the existing chemical treatments address only chemical neurotransmitter imbalances, and overlook faulty neural interconnections.

The famous but not celebrated *Diagnostic and Statistical Manual of Mental Disorders* (American Psychiatric Association 2013) has suffered many mutations and criticisms from 1952 to the present. In its current edition, the fifth, the *Manual* distinguishes about 300 mental disorders, thrice as many as in its first edition of 1952. For example, it incorporates a whole autism spectrum, and the binge-eating, hoarding, skin-picking, and persistent irritability disorders. More importantly, it has replaced the logotherapies, which have at best a placebo effect, with brain-based therapies. "In principle," though not in detail, these should handle everything mental, but so far they have not helped much to diagnose mental diseases, let alone treat them effectively. This situation is reminiscent of ancient science, which was of no use to technology.

Even after so many revisions over six decades, the *Manual* is not as well respected as other widely used and often updated medical texts, such as Cecil's *Essentials of Medicine* or Harrison's *Principles of Internal Medicine*. Why? Because the *Manual*'s diagnostic criteria are purely symptomatic — that is, superficial. Parallel: an ophthalmology manual which ignored that myopia can have many different causes: crystalline lens or cornea, retina, optical nerve, primary visual cortex, circulation, diabetes, etc. So primitive an ophthalmology could not be very effective.

The poverty of symptomatic psychiatry reached ridicule when the prestigious journal *Science* published David L. Rosenhan's (1973) "On being sane in insane places." This paper reported on a spoof practiced by Professor Rosenhan and eight healthy confederates on some of the most prestigious American psychiatric hospitals. The pseudo-patients told the hospital staff that they suffered from auditory hallucinations. They were duly diagnosed as schizophrenics, and forced to take antipsychotic drugs in accordance with the supposedly authoritative *Manual*. Some of them were even forcibly institutionalized.

When Professor Rosenhan exposed his hoax, the skeptical psychiatrists had a field day, and the anti-psychiatrist crowd ranted even more loudly against science and hospitals. No one seems to have drawn the correct methodological lesson: that a medicine relying exclusively on what patients show and tell is at best protoscientific. Scientific medicine digs for objective (biological) signs underneath subjective symptoms, because these are superficial and therefore unreliable.

A classical example is Korsakoff's dementia, clinically characterized by the inability to form new memories, amnesia, confabulation, and a lack of interest. The neural mechanism of this disease is fairly well known: Alcohol abuse $\rightarrow$ $\downarrow$ Thiamine (vitamin B1) absorption $\rightarrow$ Cell death in medial thalamus, hippocampus, and mamillary bodies $\rightarrow$ Severe loss of some mental functions. Consequently, thiamine deficiency, which can be detected through a blood analysis, is one of the objective signs (biomarkers) of Korsakoff's. Presumably, as brain-imaging methods are perfected, an early, reliable, and quick diagnosis of this incapacitating and debilitating disease will become available.

The preceding is linked with the problem of localizing the mental functions, which had occupied Galen. If the mind is immaterial, it may exist in time but not in space; otherwise it must be somewhere. Two centuries ago, the phrenologists had claimed to know exactly which functions every part of the brain performs, from desire to calculation. But their localizations were speculative, since they did not perform experiments or even autopsies to check them.

This situation changed overnight when Paul Broca in the 1860s and Karl Wernicke in 1874, localized some speech disorders, such as syntactic and semantic aphasias. Nearly one century later, Wilder Penfield and his team evoked vivid feelings and memories in waking subjects by subjecting their cerebral cortices to gentle electrical discharges at precise places. Despite his decisive contribution to the materialist view of the mind, Penfield retained the dualist doctrine he had learned as a youngster, and declined my invitation to discuss it in my seminar.

Nowadays, psychologists and psychiatrists can use three high-tech instruments — CAT, MRI, and MTI — to localize some mental processes in waking patients without operating on them. A stream of new information has thus flowed over the past three decades. MRI is also used to localize some cerebrovascular accidents, such as strokes, as well as cerebral abscesses and tumors, hence to excise them if grave. In earlier times, neurosurgeons had to operate nearly in the dark, and were confined to tumors and epileptic foci.

The invention of the above-mentioned imaging techniques was a huge advancement, because the first thing we have to learn about any fact is where and when it happens. These wondrous techniques have been ridiculed as so many attempts to revive phrenology, the discredited attempt to read the mind by palpating bumps on the skull. And yet, MRI is the only technique that yields an image of what goes on in the whole brain, and is the best tool for finding out how it develops (Bunge & Kahn 2009).

MRI has also yielded some unexpected findings, such as that (a) every stimulus to one of the senses has an echo in others; (b) the cerebellum contributes to cognition; (c) learning alters the structural connectivity of white matter, which had formerly been thought of as being unintelligent (Mackey *et al.* 2012); and (d) severe depression kills neurons galore. The MRI users hope that eventually this "cartography" will help discover well-localized mechanisms in neuronal networks, which in turn may help discover new biological psychotherapies. (See Table 4.1.)

Up to now, we have discussed only diseases that occur in isolation from others. But many disorders come in bundles or systems, which should not be surprising given that the body is a system of systems. For instance, a severe heart or kidney insufficiency will disturb nearly all the other bodily functions. Such *comorbidity* is frequent among the elderly. In these cases, the patient has several complaints at once, and his doctor must

Table 4.1. Localization of some cognitive deficits.

Damaged brain area	Cognitive deficit
Supramarginal gyrus	Apraxia
Broca area	Speech delivery
Wernicke area	Speech understanding
Mirror neurons system	"Theory" of mind
Hippocampus	Episodic memory
V4 visual area	Color vision
1st (newer) visual pathway	What is it?
2nd (older) visual pathway	Where is it?
Prefrontal cortex	Decision
Angular gyrus	Arithmetic operations

find out whether all of them have the same source, usually hidden from the patient.

A natural yet primitive reaction to such complexity is to despair of the power of analysis and proclaim the somewhat cryptic holistic slogan "The whole is greater than the sum of its parts." The scientific attitude is to insist that analysis is the more valuable the greater the complexity. But of course, a realist analysis of a whole, such as a syndrome, will distinguish its parts without detaching them from one another; it will regard them as constituents of a system, that is, an object whose parts interact with one another (recall Section 2.3).

Finally, note that our version of diagnostic reasoning involves the method of *successive approximations*, which Archimedes invented more than two millennia ago. This method involves the idea that a proposition may be more or less true or plausible. In other words, contrary to logicians but in consonance with scientific and technological practice, we suppose that there are truth values between 0 (completely false) and 1 (completely true). That is, we admit the use of *approximate truths*, such as "$\pi = 3.14$" and "The Earth is spherical" (e.g., Bunge 1967).

On the other hand, we have not admitted the idea, essential to inductive logic and Bayesian statistics, that statements can be attributed probabilities in the rigorous (mathematical) sense of the term. There are several reasons for this refusal (Bunge 2012b). One is that nobody has said what it *means* to say that "the probability of that proposition is such and such," except that probability is sometimes mistaken for degree of truth. Another reason for discarding this confusion is that, whereas physicists know how to calculate and measure the probabilities of random *facts*, neither medics nor philosophers have laid down rules for assigning probabilities to propositions. Consequently, such values are assigned arbitrarily — hardly a scientific procedure.

Nor have we found any use for *modal logic*, the set of theories about propositions of the forms "p is possible" and "p is necessary," where p names a proposition or statement. There are several reasons for not using it (Bunge 1977c). One is that modal logic is too coarse, as it does not distinguish between logical possibility (non-contradiction), epistemic (plausibility), ontological (compatibility with the relevant laws of nature), moral (fairness), technological (feasibility), and legal (compatibility with positive law). The necessity concept is parallel. For instance, biological necessity, such as that of thinking with the brain and not with the liver, has nothing to do with logical necessity (deducibility).

Another reason for avoiding modal logic is that, when dealing with real possibility, we can often use a far more potent calculus: that of probability. A third reason for not bothering with modal logic is that it encourages barren and even absurd speculations about possible worlds, notably the idea that "p is possible" amounts to "There is a parallel world, inaccessible from ours, where p is true." This is how Saul Kripke (1971) claimed to have refuted the hypothesis that the mental is cerebral; he deemed such identity untenable, since it is not *logically* necessary, for there may be worlds where people think with their feet.

A fourth reason for dispensing with modal logic is that it leads to accepting uncertainty instead of attempting to minimize it. For example, the clinician starts by juggling several possibilities but, instead of escaping to a parallel world, conducts examinations and orders tests in order to eliminate all but one of them.

In sum, medical diagnosis raises a number of interesting and tough philosophical problems. We have just dealt with one of them: that of how medics would reason if they had more logical scruples and more time. Rudolf Carnap, an exact philosopher who respected science from afar, would rightly say that ours is an example of a *rational reconstruction*. We proceed to supplementing it with an important tool: statistical control.

4.2 Statistical Control

Until recently, some medics used to boast about their "clinical eye," that is, the ability to diagnose at first sight. Thus, my father, a physician and political activist, after being questioned and threatened by the chief torturer of the day, declared confidently that the monster was so sick that he would not last six months. He was proved right, but he failed to foresee his own demise shortly thereafter.

The so-called clinical eye is a kind of intuition, or pre-analytic and fast thinking. We indulge in it when pressed for time or lacking in information. But only the intuitionist philosophers, like Henri Bergson, George E. Moore, and Edmund Husserl, have claimed that intuitions are infallible.

The rest of us have learned from bitter experience that first impressions and instant decisions are unreliable. We have learned, in fact, that appearances can be deceiving, and that sense data may motivate research but cannot replace it, because reality is stratified and the senses can only capture some traits of the upper layer. We also know that informal thinking is subject to multiple "cognitive illusions," such as the anchoring to the first datum or the first guess.

Even though philosophical analysis warns us to mistrust intuition and instant decision, we keep resorting to experts who make a good living by improvising diagnoses and prognoses: military officers, personnel chiefs, financial consultants, marriage counselors, clinical psychologists — and doctors picked from the Yellow Pages of a telephone book. Most of the judgments of these experts are based only on first impressions and very coarse estimates. Occasionally, they use objective data, such as a set of values of biomarkers, but they process them intuitively, often with the help of logical shortcuts or "heuristics," that sometimes work and other times don't. Maybe this is why Richard Feynman once said, perhaps with tongue in cheek, that "science is the belief in the ignorance of experts."

How reliable are the diagnoses and prognoses of experts who only use their experience and intuition, or who use objective data but "combine them in the head" instead of feeding them into an algorithm? The clinical psychologist and philosopher of science Paul Meehl (1954), who investigated this problem, shocked academia when he announced that the forecasts made exclusively on the basis of statistical data and "mechanical" rules are far more successful, and therefore more reliable, than the subjective or intuitive ones made by experts.

A telling example had been independently provided a year earlier by the anesthesiologist Virginia Apgar, who had proposed one of the most widely used, successful, and yet simplest of such "mechanical" rules: a checklist to assess the viability of a newborn. She proposed checking the heart rate, respiration, reflex, muscle tone, and color of the infant, and assigning each variable a value (0, 1, or 2, depending on the strength of each sign). A baby with a total score of 8 or above will make it, but one with a score of 4 or below will be in trouble, hence in urgent need of special attention.

Meehl's work was extended by his coworker Robyn Dawes (1996), and both of them joined with David Faust in writing an influential paper

(Dawes *et al.* 1989). This article provoked passionate controversy and did much to secure the prestige of the statistical approach in clinical psychology, medicine, and even the law. Psychotherapy was the main casualty of their campaign, even though Meehl was a practicing psychoanalyst. But their most important contribution is that a great many physicians now take statistics seriously when making diagnoses. (Unfortunately, they tend to call this the *Bayesian* method, which is the totally different game of pinning numbers on facts in an intuitive fashion.)

The Nobel laureate psychologist Daniel Kahneman (2011), a lifelong admirer of Meehl, and one of the earliest users of his approach to psychological diagnosis and prognosis, asked why the "clinical" or intuitive approach is far inferior to the algorithmic (or statistical, or actuarial) one. He suggested the following reasons: the clinical predictor is a victim of the halo effect; he cannot avoid being impressed by irrelevant traits; he juggles at the same time too many variables that he has no time to weigh; he is often inconsistent; and, above all, he is "overconfident in his intuitions." Clearly, algorithms do not have such flaws. (For the pros and cons of intuition, see Bunge 1962.)

Of course, statistical reasoning, in focusing on whole populations, deliberately ignores personal characteristics. Does it follow that those using statistical data to diagnose cannot prescribe a treatment tailored to the patient's peculiarities? Yes, if they use only statistics; no, if they also use personal data, such as age, family antecedents, surgeries, allergies, occupation, and recent relevant incidents. And this is, precisely, what all physicians and nurses do: to them, every patient is unique in several respects. All medicines have always been tailored, even though "personalization," that is, therapy tailored to the individual genome, is a very recent development.

Here is an instructive case. Emile Durkheim, one of the fathers of modern sociology, became famous overnight in 1897 for announcing that Protestants commit suicide far more frequently than Catholics. He concluded this by examining a great number of death certificates; whereas those of the Catholic suicides state that they had died of heart attack, those of the Protestant suicides were veridical. This difference made sense: suicide is a mortal sin according to Catholic doctrine, not so according to Protestantism.

Nearly a century later, it was found that the signatories of the Catholic certificates had committed pious lies to save the face of the suicides' families. Presumably, a comparison of the cardiopathy statistics would have exposed the inoffensive fraud. A more recent and relevant case is the abnormally high frequency of heart attacks among political prisoners, compared with the corresponding frequency in the general population.

There is a consensus that statistics are indispensable to know and manage populations of all kinds, since they teach how to produce statistical parameters, such as averages, medians, and variances, in large scale. But, as Claude Bernard noted long ago, statistics do not yield substantive knowledge, because they do not study things but only selected data about them. For example, statistics help process data about the body mass index (weight in kilograms/square of height in meters), but it does not explain why this indicator has been rising so quickly in recent years in the West, nor why it is the lowest in Japan and Korea. Statistical data may *pose* research problems, such as looking for causation underneath correlation, but they do not solve them.

It is sometimes objected that sticking to guidelines of any kind, in particular subjecting new therapies to randomized controlled trials, slows down clinical decision-making, when the physician's personal experience should suffice. This objection overlooks the importance of the quality of the decision. One also saves time by estimating distances and times instead of measuring them, but that does not work for regulating air traffic. Instant medical diagnoses are justified in the emergency room, but they are only preliminary and subject to revision.

Let us finally glance at the leap from statistical correlation to causation. We begin by recalling the classical criteria proposed by Austin Bradford Hill (1965), the eminent biostatistician who designed the first randomized controlled trial (for streptomycin) and who, along with the epidemiologist Robert Doll, proved that cigarette smoking causes lung cancer. Here are Bradford Hill's conditions for inferring causation from statistical association:

1) strong statistical correlation;
2) consistency (in different populations and under different circumstances);
3) specificity (a single effect);
4) antecedence (the presumed cause must precede the effect);

5) biological gradient (the magnitude of the effect increases with that of the cause);
6) biological plausibility (mechanism of action);
7) coherence with the rest of the relevant information;
8) experimental proof; and
9) analogy.

By itself, none of these nine factors is sufficient or even necessary; Bradford Hill's idea was that the conjunction of all of them was both necessary and sufficient to conjecture causation. But he admitted that this conjecture is not conclusive.

I suggest keeping only the *specificity, antecedence, plausibility, coherence* (or *external consistency*), and *experimental proof* conditions. The last involves the biological gradient condition, since experiment will show what happens when the cause (e.g., the dose) is altered. Experiment and plausibility also render strong correlation redundant; its only role is heuristic. The consistency requirement is excessive, since every population contains individuals who are much less susceptible than others, perhaps because they have been immunized. Finally, we should not require analogy, because there is always some similarity with something else. In sum, statistical data may suggest causal hypotheses. When they do, those data are best forgotten, and a new research project is to be planned: that of subjecting those hypotheses to further experimental tests.

In sum, statistics is a heuristic tool for diagnosis. In turn, reliable statistics depend critically on correct diagnosis. However, we must face the following paradox. A decrease in the rate of a disease may be attributed to improvements in either health care or lifesyle. But an increase in the said rate may be due to a diagnostic advance — to the fact that new diagnostic tools have made it possible to detect ailments that had previously escaped the physicians' notice. (This may explain the current trend in cancer rates; while breast and lung cancers are decreasing, pancreatic and kidney cancers seem to be on the rise.) The moral of this story is, of course, that data are just as fallible as hypotheses. Only objective facts are "hard." This moral shows, once more, the superiority of realism over empiricism.

4.3 The Probabilistic Siren

Statistics and statistical theory are about *collections* of things or facts, such as human populations and sets of gunshot victims. In particular, epidemiological statistics exhibit the frequencies with which diseases occur in different populations. Frequencies, along with averages and variances, are *collective properties*, and they are extracted from data concerning the individuals constituting the population in question — for instance, by counting the victims of a plague. Hence, those statistical data do not tell us anything about the individuals concerned, except that they have the traits that are being investigated, as well as that such traits are rare or, on the contrary, rather common.

By contrast, probabilities are properties of *individual* facts. For example, one may speak of the probability that an American selected at random is addicted to a hard drug. Note the word *random*. The idea is that *talk of probability is justified only when there is chance*, and conversely so (Humphreys 1985; Bunge 2006). Chance may be in things (e.g., atoms) or in the sampling of a population (e.g., when persons are allotted blindly to the experimental and control groups in an experiment). In either case, probabilities are objective; they are properties of things and events out there, not of beliefs.

Furthermore, the probability concept is theoretical, not empirical like that of frequency, i.e., probabilities are assumed or calculated, never directly measured. True, we often talk about intuitively *estimating* the probabilities of certain events, much in the same way that we estimate ages or weights. But we usually do so knowing that they are approximate and corrigible values.

Whether probabilities are postulated, calculated, or merely guessed, how are they checked? The answer depends on the type of random fact and on the relevant theory. The simplest case is that of a mass of equally probable alternatives whose frequencies can be counted, as in games of chance and in the sex of human fetuses. For example, the probability that a fetus is a girl is 0.5 because meiosis — the process of the combination of the parents' genomes — is objectively random. But, once the egg has been fertilized, probability vanishes: the child will be either a girl or a boy. Probability reappears only if an individual is picked at random (with blindfold) from a large

Table 4.2. The proper places of the most outstanding members of the randomness family. The statistical parameters are measurable, and can also be calculated from a probability distribution.

Reality	Theory	Observation or experiment
Chance	Probability	Frequency, average, variance

human population — provided there has been no girl infanticide. In sum, after zygote formation, sex is no longer a random variable. (See Table 4.2.)

It is sometimes said that causation obtains when probability equals 1. There are even probabilistic theories of causation. But the concepts of causation and probability are mutually independent; they are not interdefinable. Indeed, the former is ontological whereas the latter is mathematical, even though it may be interpreted as the measure of the possibility of a random fact. Causation obtains only when there is an energy gradient, and there is objective probability when there is more than one real possibility. Yet, although the two concepts are not interdefinable, they can be related, namely thus: if C and E are random facts, and C causes E, then the (conditional) probability of E given C is greater than the (unconditional) probability of E: $P(E|C) \geq P(E)$.

The reverse leap, from probability to causality, is fallacious, if only because causality involves reference to energy or even mechanism, which probability does not. However, such a leap is a fertile heuristic strategy; if one finds that fact C favors (probabilifies) the occurrence of fact E, then one may suspect that maybe C is a (not *the*) cause of E.

For example, one is more likely to "catch" a cold during the flu season, when "the bug is going around," than during the summer, and contagion may happen through a chance encounter with someone who sneezes without covering her mouth. In this case, chance is in the encounter, not in the rhinovirus spread by the sick individual. (Much the same holds for the hypothesis of random mating.) Only the unveiling of a mechanism may confirm or refute a causal guess. Randomness guesses are parallel; only the presence of a randomizer, such as blind shuffling or agitation (as in heating) justifies talk of chance, hence of probability.

The preceding refers to the manner in which the probability concept is used in the so-called hard sciences. Elsewhere, the word 'probability' is sometimes used as a synonym for the *intensity of a belief.* This is the *subjective* or *Bayesian* interpretation, a darling of philosophers, and that has appeared with increasing frequency in the medical literature since about 1980 (e.g., Wulff 1981). However, some medics misuse 'probability' as a synonym of 'frequency,' and 'Bayesian' for 'statistical.'

The authentic Bayesian allots the probability values he wishes, and he does not mind if different persons assign different probabilities to the same events; Bayesian probabilities are as subjective as aesthetic preferences. Bruno de Finetti (1972), their modern prophet, called them *personal.* This view has suggested the famous cartoon where the doctor tells his patient that his staff estimates that there is a 70% probability of heart failure, and a 15% probability that they know what they are talking about.

The concepts of objective chance (or disorder), randomization, and objective or impersonal probability do not occur in the Bayesian literature. Nor does that of personal probability occur in physics, chemistry, or biology. Because personal probability is arbitrary, it has no place in science, engineering, or scientific medicine (Bunge 2008). Yet, it is often used, even in drug trials, because it saves brain work, time, and money, as will be seen in Chapter 6. The example to be discussed next should show the absurdity and danger of the Bayesian approach to disease, etiology, and therapy.

It is well known that HIV infection is a necessary cause of AIDS: no HIV, no AIDS. In other words, having AIDS implies having HIV, though not the converse. Suppose now that a given individual b has been proved to be HIV-positive. A Bayesian will ask what is the probability that b has or will eventually develop AIDS. To answer this question, the Bayesian assumes that the Bayes' theorem applies, and writes down this formula: $P(\text{AIDS} | \text{HIV}) = P(\text{HIV} | \text{AIDS}) \cdot P(\text{AIDS})/P(\text{HIV})$, where an expression of the form $P(A)$ means the absolute (or prior) probability of A in the given population, whereas $P(A | B)$ is read (or interpreted) as "the conditional probability of A given (or assuming) B."

If the lab analysis shows that b carries the HIV, the Bayesian will set $P(\text{HIV}) = 1$. And, since all AIDS patients are HIV carriers, he will also set $P(\text{HIV} | \text{AIDS}) = 1$. Substituting these values into Bayes' formula yields $P(\text{AIDS} | \text{HIV}) = P(\text{AIDS})$. But this result is false, since there are persons with HIV but no AIDS. What is the source of this error? It comes from assuming tacitly that carrying HIV and suffering from AIDS are random facts, hence subject to probability theory. The HIV–AIDS connection is causal, not casual; HIV infection is only a necessary cause of AIDS. In conclusion, contrary to what Bayesians (and rational-choice theorists) assume, it is wrong to assign probabilities to all facts. Only random facts, as well as facts picked at random, have probabilities.

A lesson of the foregoing for medical diagnosis is that phrases of the form "The probability that this patient suffers from disease X" are wrong, because getting sick is a causal event, not a random one — not even when the disease has been caught in a chance encounter. Health care workers examine people who either suffer from a given disease or not. Likewise, it makes no sense to wonder about the probability that our next-door neighbor is the nation's president, because this job is not won in a raffle. Chance is for real but not ever-present. If it were, medics would be no better than gamblers. (See additional criticisms in Eddy & Clanton 1982; Murphy 1997.) Moreover, if the medics who take Bayes' formula seriously were consistent, they would have to admit the possibility of resurrection, since the mindless application of the said formula allows one to calculate the probability $P(A|D)$ of being alive after dying, from the inverse probability $P(D|A)$ of dying and the absolute probabilities or priors $P(A)$ of being alive, and $P(D)$ of being dead.

The Bayesian or subjective probabilities are popular outside the "hard" sciences precisely because they are not rigorous; they allow anyone to fill pages with exact formulas impregnable to empirical test because they just express personal beliefs. For example, in their rather popular biostatistics manual, Berry and Stangl (1996: 8) write that the Bayesian interpretation fits the health sciences because, in these, differences of opinion are the norm. Fortunately, the responsible doctor and the thoughtful patient will beg to differ; they will ask for a second opinion, or even for a panel of experts, of whom one expects not just opinion but argument based on scientific knowledge. The ancient Greeks made much of the difference between *episteme* or science and *doxa* or opinion. The postmoderns deny this difference, but the rest of us have kept it because we care for truth and well-grounded action.

Coda

Why do so many diagnoses prove wrong? First, because although anyone can diagnose, correct diagnosis is an objectively hard task. Why? Because it is an inverse problem, of the Effect → Cause type, rather than a direct one. And there are no algorithms ("mechanical rules") for solving inverse problems, just as there are no algorithms for inventing new ideas. In science and technology, to handle an inverse problem, one must invent and try out conjectures — though not arbitrary ones but only hypotheses compatible with the bulk of antecedent knowledge.

Yet, there is a general strategy to approach inverse problems, namely to transform them into direct ones. This is done by investigating the mechanism of the process in question. When that factor and only that one is found to be "responsible" for this medical sign, one has hit on the correct diagnosis. For example, only the increasing fibrosis of the bone marrow and its consequent progressive failure to produce blood explain the monotonous decrease in red blood cells and the eventual onset of anemia and ultimately leukemia: the case of myelofibrosis.

If, by contrast, the physician confines himself to symptoms, as still happens routinely in the case of mental disorders, diagnosis becomes a hit-and-miss game, since almost any mental symptom, from confusion and amnesia to delusion and depression, may be due to many different causes. This is why the progress of medicine, which accompanies the enrichment of the battery of objective signs or biomarkers concomitant with the discovery of mechanisms, depends critically on basic research.

The search for mechanisms of action is encouraged by philosophical realism, which is at variance with the phenomenalism (or sticking to appearances) inherent in empiricism from Ptolemy to Hume to Comte to Mach to Carnap. However, modern medicine requires empirical verification — the saving grace of empiricism and the ogre of "alternative" medicine. Medical diagnosis will always be fallible but also corrigible, sometimes even in time, as long as medicine keeps it scientific roots, but it may never become certain.

It has been said that probability quantifies uncertainty and, since medicine is an uncertain art, its practitioners should reason in probabilistic terms. But this view is doubly erroneous. First, because disease and treatment are causal processes, not random ones. For instance, you either have a cold or don't, so that it is not legitimate to ask what is the probability that you are nursing a cold. Second, because medicine does not contain any important probabilistic theories. (Only these contain an objective measure of uncertainty, namely the variance or spread of a distribution such as a scatter plot.)

The case of statistics is very different. It is proper and convenient to use statistical data in framing diagnoses and prognoses, because they contain valuable heuristic pointers. For example, since diabetes is frequent among the Inuit, the doctors attending members of that ethnic group are advised to start by conducting diabetes tests. But they would not be justified in mistaking such frequencies for probabilities and in using Bayes' theorem to make diagnoses, for becoming diabetic is a causal process.

In sum, diagnosis is and will always be a central, interesting, and far from trivial conceptual task for medics. Consequently, it should draw the attention of philosophers. Sadly, though, none of the best-known philosophers has handled this problem — which speaks to the problematic relevance of academic philosophy to real life.

CHAPTER 5

DRUG

5.1 Classical Pharmacology

In 1892, when William Osler's classical treatise on medicine appeared, every well-educated Western European physician was confident that he could correctly diagnose any ailment except perhaps for tropical diseases. But Osler felt exasperated because he was nearly impotent to cure most of them. For this reason, he always carried morphine in his doctor's bag. The reason for his exasperation was the dearth of effective drugs and vaccines at his disposal.

At that time, there were only two well-tried treatments: bed rest, which used to be unnecessarily long, and surgery, which was not always safe. There were also only two vaccines — against smallpox and rabies — as well as a dozen useful drugs, among them phenol (disinfectant), iodine (to disinfect and against goiter), sodium bicarbonate (against acid reflux), quinine and artemisine (both to control malarial fevers), and opiates (analgesics and hypnotics).

Some of the most popular medical drugs were ineffective and others, such as the arsenic and mercury compounds, were toxic. Osler was so skeptical about the pharmacopeia of his time, that he was accused of "therapeutic nihilism" (Bliss 1999). Actually, Osler was not a nihilist but a skeptic, and not a radical one, since he spent much of his legendary energy improving medical education on the basis of the biomedical sciences, which had been advancing rapidly since the 1850s.

Drug penury started to change toward the end of the nineteenth century, with the quick development of scientific pharmacology and large-scale pharma industry, especially in Germany. That industry started spectacularly with the synthesis and large-scale manufacture of "the drug of the century" — acetylsalicylic acid, or aspirin (1899). This rather simple molecule ($C_9H_8O_4$) resulted from adding five atoms to that of salicylic acid, which had adverse effects. Another sensational triumph of the new industry was Salvarsan (1910), the first effective and humane drug against syphilis. The third amazing invention was that of insulin (1922). Only one decade later, Prontosil (sulfamidocrisoidine), the first antibiotic, reached the market. Three of those four "wonder drugs" were synthesized — the first wholly artificial medical drugs.

Since then, the pharmacopeia in the prosperous nations has gone from a dozen to a thousand standard remedies. About 50 new medical drugs enter the market every year. One may expect that the number of drugs will keep increasing as chemists and pharmacologists synthesize molecules of new species and find new therapeutic uses for known molecules. However, we must also consider the narrow economic interest of the pharma industry.

In the entire history of the universe, there may not have been as creative a power as modern pharmacology. But the yield of searches for new molecular species is very low: 96% of them lasted only the few minutes it took a machine to check their medical potential. Besides, this wealthy pharmacopeia is accessible to only two of every seven fellow humans. Furthermore, the pharma industry tends to produce only highly profitable drugs; it is conservative, while pharmacology is revolutionary.

The alphabetical list of the drugs available in the market contains 40 names of drugs between Aa and Ac. But 90% of the sales at Western pharmacies are reduced to only 10 drugs, and 40% to three kinds: antacids, anti-cholesterols, and antidepressants.

Ten percent of the health budget of the prosperous nations is spent on medical drugs. About $100 billion per year are invested worldwide in drug research and development. However, almost the entirety of this task is being performed in universities and state research institutes such as the National Institutes of Health, at taxpayers' expense. But only 10% of this budget is devoted to studying drugs to treat diseases typical of the underdeveloped nations: parasitoses of various kinds, tuberculosis, malaria, Chagas disease, and dengue fever. There are, then, two pharmacopeias: one for the rich and another for the poor.

Still, there has been sensational progress, to the point that most of us have come to believe the formula *a pill for every ill*. Consequently, selling medical drugs has become as lucrative as selling arms or narcotics. But this

not made friends for either pharmacology or the pharma indus-
contrary, we are witnessing a cultural backlash — the indigna-
by the disproportionate price of medical drugs and the reluctance
rma to manufacture generics (at one-third the price of brand
been compounded by the resentment that scientific and techno-
ncements provoke among those who are left behind for lack of
education. This second motive explains why the enemies of
concentrated in churches and humanities departments.

n against cultural innovation is not new. The ancient
an world was destroyed not only by barbarian invaders, but
destructive frenzy of the masses that had been left outside the
ure; they adopted exotic religions, like Christianity and
that were hostile to learning and the arts; the seventeenth-
ch Craze followed in the wake of the Scientific Revolution;
philosophies of Kant and Hegel reacted against the materialism
n of the radical wing of the French Enlightenment; psychoa-
tionism, phenomenology, existentialism, linguistic philosophy,
c Marxism became popular at the same time that atomic phys-
ry, pharmacology, neuroscience, evolutionary biology, and
nd rigorous disciplines flourished.

gards demonized the science that they could not understand
tradicted their unexamined beliefs. And they were often
lf-styled leftists incapable of distinguishing knowledge from
by those who imagined that medicine is just a tool of the
cal industry; and by those who wish to judge science with
eria instead of engaging in the much harder task of thinking
olitics with the help of science. In sum, it would seem that
cal theorem about the reaction provoked by every action
n the realm of culture. However, it is time to go back to
gy.

pharmacology, the science and technology of the medically
ecules, emerged from two successive mergers:

〉 *Biochemistry*
ry   〉
                                    Scientific pharmacology

In turn, the history of scientific pharmacology consists of two stages: classical and molecular. The classical pharmacologists engaged in applied analytical chemistry: they analyzed natural products, mostly vegetal, in order to isolate their presumed therapeutic constituents. For example, in 1828, willow bark, known as an analgesic since antiquity, was analyzed to isolate its "active principle"; the result was salicine, from which salicylic acid ($C_8H_7O_2COOH$) was extracted. This turned out to be a good pain-killer, but also a gastric irritant. To neutralize its acidity, it was combined wih a buffer, until in 1899, aspirin — the first synthetic drug — flooded the world market.

The history of aspirin is normal in modern experimental science and medicine:

Background knowledge → *Problem* → *Research project* → *Hypothesis*
→ *Partially successful trial* → *New hypothesis* → *New trial* → . . .

This version of the scientific method differs from the empiricist version found in most textbooks: *Observation* → *Hypothesis* → *Prediction* → *Trial*. It also differs from Popper's refutationist one:

Myth → *Refutation* → *Hypothesis* → *Trial* → *Refutation* → *New hypothesis* → . . .

Empiricism makes us mistrust uncontrolled speculation, but it also inhibits us from digging beneath the tangible. And refutationism provokes us like Tantalus, but does not allow us to reach for truths, and thus counsels radical skepticism — the view that there are no final truths.

If Louis Pasteur had been an empiricist, he would not have speculated about microbes, and he would not have suspected that pristine black soil is chock-full of bacteria, among them the deadly tetanus and anthrax. And if he had been a refutationist, Pasteur would have remained content with refuting the myth of the spontaneous and sudden emergence of multicellular organisms from river mud.

Fortunately, Pasteur knew intuitively that, as Heraclitus had said, "nature likes to hide," so that one should dig beneath the data (e.g., infection points to bacteria). But he might not have adopted this stance before the invention of the microscope, the earliest and most powerful anti-empiricist instrument — though one that failed to discourage the phenomenalist philosophers, for whom only appearances count.

Pasteur also knew that the goal of scientific research is not to bury ideas but to cultivate them. His research also exemplifies the difference between seeking to confirm a conjecture and trying to falsify it. Indeed, when Pasteur sought to corroborate the microbe hypothesis, he protected them from possible contamination, but when intent on refuting the spontaneous generation legend, he boiled them to death. Incidentally, contrary to legend, Pasteur did not dash the materialist hypothesis of the abiotic origin of life; he only proved the impossibility of the emergence of ready-made multicellular organisms from non-living matter. In fact, Oparin's (1924) project of synthesizing cells in the laboratory (abiogenesis) is alive and well, as a glance at the recent literature (e.g., Luisi 2006; Lazcano 2007) will confirm.

5.2 Molecular Pharmacology

Pharmacologists have always tackled problems of two kinds: *direct* (or Cause → Effect) problems, such as finding out the effects of alleged remedies on an organism, and *inverse* (or Effect → Cause) problems, those of finding or designing drugs with the desired effects. Obviously, the inverse problems, those of meeting demands, call for much more practical imagination than the direct ones of analyzing given products. It is not so much that studying the given is easier than imagining what there might be, but that the two tasks require skills of very different kinds.

The classical pharmacologists confined themselves to studying and trying out medically promising natural products. By contrast, the molecular pharmacologists design and build new molecules, the vast majority of which do not exist in nature. And, since a designed molecule is an artifact, its designer is a technologist. Hence, molecular pharmacology is sandwiched between basic science and technology. We shall return to this subject in Chapter 10.

Whereas sane laymen avoid known toxics, pharmacologists seek to transform some of them into medical drugs. The reason is that most toxics are synthesized by organisms. In fact, some of the toxics utilizable in this manner are the defenses of certain plants against predators. For example, some drugs used as antihypertensives or to treat cardiac insufficiency originate from the poison of a Brazilian snake. (Who knows what useful drugs may result from the pharmacology of human endotoxins, or what antibodies might be discovered by studying bats, which are hosts of the Ebola, SARS, and other dreadful viruses that do not seem to sicken them?) Furthermore, the study of the coevolution of plants and animals — for example, the seeds eaten and spread by birds — may yield findings of interest to pharmacology.

The study of what a drug does in the body (i.e., drug metabolism) is disinterested, but the concern for how well the patient who took the drug is doing is far from disinterested. In short, the study of drugs and the treatments involving them goes back and forth between basic science and technology — a characteristic of applied science. Two flows at once distinguish and join the three fields in question: basic science feeds knowledge to both applied science and technology, which in turn pose problems to the former:

Technology
Knowledge ↑ Applied science ↓ *Problems*
Basic science

Marie Curie, who won two Nobel Prizes for her research in basic physics, noted that disinterested research may yield unexpected practical fruits, such as the medical use of radioisotopes. It has been estimated that 80% of the increase in the GDP of the advanced nations during the last century was ultimately due to basic research. This datum should suffice to indict the myopic science policies that require immediate practical results from people who are unable to produce them because they trained to explore reality, not to alter it. In short, pragmatism is impractical.

As noted in the previous section, the classical pharmacologists extracted drugs from natural products. From the mid-nineteenth century on, some pharmacologists chose a harder path: they started from comparatively simple molecules and combined them with others to obtain more complex molecules with possible therapeutic properties. The ulterior preclinical trial, in the laboratory or on animal "models," may tell whether in fact they have such desirable traits. But before starting such time-consuming trials, researchers study in detail the complicated metabolism of the potential drug, from its absorption by the liver or the intestine to its excretion by the kidneys. (Actually, the pronoun 'its' is out of place here, because the metabolism of a drug involves transformations of the intake into a sequence of different metabolites.)

Moreover, researchers also attempt to find out the mechanisms of the action of the drug and its metabolites. These mechanisms are chemical reactions, such as oxidation, which are catalyzed by enzymes called P450 cytochromes, of which there are thousands of types. Presumably, if all these had been designed intelligently, the metabolism of drugs and foods would be far simpler, faster, and more energy-efficient. (For one thing, there would be no toxic metabolites.) But biological evolution is notoriously opportunistic, slow, and wasteful.

Although the preceding may suggest that pharmacology is nothing but applied chemistry, in fact it is no such thing, because it makes intensive use of anatomy, physiology, cellular biology, bacteriology, and virology, in addition to molecular biology — and, above all, disciplined imagination. For example, the design of antiviral drugs requires a lot of knowledge about viruses and the cells that host them, as well as about the genes they penetrate and mutate. The first thing that must be known about viruses is that they are not independent organisms but parasites, so that any drug that harms them may also harm their hosts. Moreover, they cannot be killed because they are not alive, but they can be disabled or even dismantled.

This is why any successful attack on viruses won't be frontal, but will target the components of a cell required for the virus' replication. A coarse military analog is the bombing of the enemy's supply sources. This pharmacological strategy is one more proof that molecular pharmacology, unlike its classical predecessor, is not a trial-and-error endeavor — except when both the assembly and the trial of new drugs are done by machines.

Still, although drug design is rational, it is not infallible. To hit its target, it must not only devise the correct molecular configuration, but also the right pharmacodynamic action. That is, the effect of the artificial molecule on the cell target must be guessed correctly. A famous and yet fertile error in the long run was designing the AZT drug assuming that all cancers are caused by viruses. AZT did not hit the original target because cancers are not caused by viruses, but it proved effective to treat AIDS, which is caused by the HIV. Any LEGO player will understand this.

The rational design of drugs is the opposite of trial and error. But this blind procedure reappears in the "translation" processes, that is, when going from the laboratory to the large-scale search for the selection, production, and pretrial of new molecules. In fact, more than 10 million molecular species are known, and every day many new ones are discovered by combining simpler molecules more or less at random: this is what combinatorial chemistry is about.

These operations are performed by robots that work without pause and, on top of making new molecules, find out whether these have any effects on cells or tissues. (Thus, they *discover* new things, whereas their designers were *inventors*.) Such automation of pharmacodynamic screening amounts to millions of experiments per year. It would take nature many millions of years to do anything like that.

The few molecules that pass those laboratory tests are subjected to preclinical tests, that is, they are tested on lab animals. If found effective, the assays are repeated on volunteers who hire out their bodies as if they were renting houses, except that they are not always warned of all the risks they take. We shall glance at this moral problem in Chapter 9.

Once again, the preceding may give the impression that, when absorbed by megaindustry, pharmacology uses brains only to design machines and computer programs, as well as marketing strategies. A glance at the most advanced stage of that technoscience will show that such impression is superficial. Indeed, the pharmacologist's goal is to engage in drug design starting from some knowledge of receptors, in the manner that tailors design made-to-measure clothes rather than in accordance with standard patterns designed by using data found by anthropologists. Their optimistic slogan is, to paraphrase Archimedes', *Give me a receptor and I'll design the molecule that will activate it*, either stimulating or blocking it (see Katzung *et al.* 2007).

As we saw in Chapter 1, the chemical receptors in organisms are large molecules, mostly proteins, attached to cell membranes. They either sit on the membrane, or are deeply rooted on it, i.e., the transmembrane receptors. In either case, receptors, like all molecules, are highly selective; they respond only to foreign molecules of certain kinds. In turn, a receptor's response activates or inhibits a cell process in a specific manner, such as contraction or division.

A drug that binds with a receptor and activates it is called an *agonist*, while an *antagonist* prevents the access of other molecules by binding with the receptor. The β blockers, some of the most effective of all synthetic drugs, act by attaching to certain proteins in the heart cells, protecting them from epinephrine (adrenaline), a potent heart excitant. Another powerful antagonist is the antiretroviral drug that blocks HIV from binding with cells. In both cases, the "stimulus" — the drug — does not stimulate but protects, as it averts the intervention of harmful inputs.

A drug that acts on receptors of a single type is called "clean." The "dirty" drugs, by contrast, act on receptors of more than one kind, and consequently have side effects, some of them neutral but others adverse. For example, most antihistamines double as sleeping pills. The great majority of the constituents of the primitive and traditional pharmacopeias were very "dirty." A goal of drug design is to get ever better-targeted compounds.

Obviously, the molecular design of drugs requires the assistance of cellular biologists interested in discovering and studying detectors. And, since there are only a couple of thousand detector types, it is likely that there will never be more than a couple of thousand basic or "clean" pharmaceutical drugs.

Now, since receptors are proteins, and since protein synthesis is guided by nucleic acids, it is necessary to go down to their level. This feature doubles the philosophical interest of drug design, for it is a two-tier inverse problem (DNA → receptor → drug), the solution to which requires descending to the molecular root of diseases and drugs. The difficulty of this task may be guessed from the fact that the way insulin binds to its receptor was uncovered 90 years after the former's isolation.

In any event, present-day pharmacology is far ahead of its classical precursor, which did not reach the molecular level and proceeded by trial and error. Presumably, all the modern philosophers, with the exception of d'Holbach and his materialist friends — notably Diderot, Helvétius, and La Mettrie — would have denounced molecular pharmacology for daring to go beyond phenomena (appearances). For better or for worse, pharmacologists are indifferent to philosophy even while practicing it.

We have come a long way from the popular or empiricist methodology of science, which demands starting always from observations and never

losing touch with them. We are also rather far from Popper's refutationism, which claims that the origin and plausibility of hypotheses makes no
difference: that only their refutability matters. We claim that the content
or pedigree of hypotheses is important too: because time and resources are
scarce, no one has enough of either to test guesses that are wildly at variance with the bulk of antecedent scientific knowledge.

In particular, the pharmacologist who uses expensive laboratory equipment, and is assisted by technicians and graduate students, cannot risk trying
out novel ideas totally lacking in chemical or biological support. He
requires, on the contrary, that the hypotheses he handles enjoy what may
be called *external consistency*, that is, plausibility in light of the best relevant
knowledge (Bunge 1967). For instance, if an enthusiast of a natural product,
such as chamomile, claims that it should be tried out, the scientist is likely
to reply: Be my guest, since the *onus probandi*, or burden of proof, rests on
the proposer. Incidentally, this is one of the classical rules of rational debate.

Any contemporary debate on the mental should include a discussion of
drugs that alter mental processes. These should be of great interest to philosophers, since their mere existence confutes the traditional view of the
mind as an immaterial entity. Indeed, if minds were souls, our reasoning
should be impregnable to the common-cold virus as well as to alcohol,
coffee, Valium, Prozac, and even heroin. The powerful psychoneuropharmaceutical industry rests on psychoneuroscience, which in turn was cued
by the old materialist hypothesis that the mental is cerebral. Yet, none of
the most popular philosophers of mind — Noam Chomsky, Jaegwon Kim,
Hilary Putnam, and Saul Kripke — has tackled this problem. They prefer
to fantasize about innate knowledge, zombies (mindless humans), or parallel worlds (such as a dry Earth).

The mind-boggling psychoneuropharmaceutical industry faced a crisis
in 2011, when nearly all the firms in this industry gave up brain research
because it was yielding diminishing returns. In particular, the clinical trials
of drugs for treating deep depression, and for repairing the harm done by
cerebrovascular accidents, failed to yield positive results. The reason is that
the new psychotropic drugs were not new enough; there were just minor
tweaks on the ones discovered half a century earlier.

Schwab and Buchli (2012) regretted that this corporate decision was
taken just at the moment when "the antiquated view of the central nervous

system as a hard-wired supercomputer has been overturned: the brain and spinal cord now appear as dynamic and adaptable biological systems." The human brain is so plastic, that Ramachandran (2011) has proposed renaming our species *Homo plasticus*. (The neural plasticity hypothesis was the axis of the theory of mind in Bunge 1980.)

The medical reason for keeping up brain research is of course that the design and trial of drugs capable of repairing "insults" to nervous tissue are based on research about neural plasticity. And the political reason for furthering such research is that the care of brain patients is costing more than that demanded by cancer, cardiovascular, and diabetes patients combined. However, back to the superiority of molecular over classical pharmacology.

Classical pharmacologists treated both medical drugs and their targets — organs and their cellular components — as *black boxes* (or input–output devices). By contrast, their successors analyze them at the molecular level, hence as *translucent boxes*. In particular, they seek to design drugs that attack cancerous cells by controlling their DNA in such a way that it inhibits some of their essential properties, notably cell division — for, unless checked at its source, the process culminates in malignant tumors.

The transition from black boxes to translucent boxes is not peculiar to pharmacology; it has occurred in all the sciences since about 1800, and it happened behind the back of most philosophers, who remained stuck in phenomenalism. Those transitions have been doubly innovating. First, the unveiling of mechanisms is accompanied by a shift from description to explanation. Second, by manipulating mechanisms, science provides technology with tools to design two-tier artifacts, micro and macro. For example, the lucrative antacid industry exploits knowledge about the neutralization of hydrochloric acid in the stomach. Thus, sodium bicarbonate — the oldest, most versatile, most popular, and cheapest of these remedies — acts thus: it combines with hydrochloric acid, producing common salt and carbonic acid, which in turn dissociates into water and carbon dioxide.

The vast majority of the chemical reactions that keep organisms alive are much more complex and faster than the neutralization of stomach acid. For one thing, they involve enzymes. These are proteins, large molecules that catalyze chemical reactions; they accelerate or even make them possible. They are highly specific (one enzyme, one chemical reaction) and the most efficient workers known; some of the 10,000 enzymes in the human cell convert millions of substrate molecules per minute. Arthur Kornberg (1989: 36), who devoted his life to studying enzymes, rhapsodized that they are "what gives the cell its life and personality."

What is a catalyzer's mechanism of action? Over decades, chemists stuck to the observation that catalyzers reappear unscathed among the reaction products, so that they seemed to act by their mere presence. The "witness" hypothesis, though satisfactory to an empiricist, seemed a matter of magic. In 1913, Leonor Michaelis and Maud Menten suggested that catalyzers participate actively in reactions. For example, if A and B name two substances without mutual affinity, the chemist may ask what would happen if a suitable catalyzer C were added. With insight, experience, or luck, the scientist will choose a C that combines transitorily with the substrate A, forming the transient compound AC, which in turn will combine with the substrate B, with the end result $AB + C$. This outcome meets the need to understand, and it suggests replacing C with an even more suitable one — faster, cheaper, or less contaminating. (Note the ambiguity of chemical notation: in the foregoing, capital letters name chemical species, but actually only individual members of those species enter into chemical reactions, see Bunge 1979.)

There is much more: when the catalyzer is an enzyme, as in nearly all biochemical reactions, it combines with a substrate in a manner reminiscent of the way in which a key fits a lock. This is the lock-and-key mechanism first proposed by Emil Fischer in 1894. Daniel Koshland refined this model in 1958, by conceiving of enzymes as flexible ("floppy") bodies with a rapidly variable geometric shape. Since then, it became clear that the shape of molecules is not only a product of internal forces and external constraints, but that it may also have causal power. Aristotle, who invented the concept of formal cause, might have felt vindicated.

Pharmacologists are just as scientific as chemists or biologists, but usually they are not driven by disinterested curiosity; instead, they focus on things and processes of *possible* utility or disutility to the health of organisms. (Note that the value concept, absent from physics and chemistry, is central to biology and biomedical science, for there are facts that are good for health and others that are bad for it.) The processes in question are the myriad chemical reactions that occur simultaneously in any organism and at various levels. Pharmacologists study them so as to control them for the good of the organism.

This study requires today much more than test tubes, pipettes, scales, and spectrographs, because of the tiny quantities of reactants and the very high speed of chemical reactions, which may not last more than a few hundreds of femtoseconds. (One femtosecond is the 10^{-15}th part of a second. A retina pigment takes about 200 femtoseconds to react to light.) A moral of this story is that the progress of pharmacology depends on that of many disciplines. In general, science is a system that does not function well unless all its components prosper.

The most successful pharmacological projects are of course those that yield new medical drugs that have passed rigorous clinical trials — the subject of the next chapter. The typical dose of a prescription drug is of a few milligrams, and it is composed of atoms, such as those of lithium, potassium, and calcium, or of small molecules consisting of 10 to 100 atoms, whereas the proteins they interact with are combinations of several thousand atoms. For example, the formula of the potent Prozac molecule is $C_{17}H_{18}F_3NO$.

This molecule should not be imagined as a conglomerate of 40 atoms because, when two or more atoms combine, they lose their individuality, for their elementary constituents are radically reorganized. The same holds, a fortiori, for large molecules such as proteins, hormones, and antibodies, with molecular weights between 5,000 and 70,000 or even more. True, molecules are usually pictured as balls joined by rods, but this is nothing but a crude classical analog. The atoms of a molecule are not its *constituents* but its *precursors*, much as a person's genome is not the sum of her parents' genomes. Chemical combination has fascinated philosophers as different as Hegel and Stuart Mill, because it is a typical instance of *emergence*, or occurrence of qualitative novelty; the products of a chemical reaction possess properties that their precursors, the reagents, do not.

As we saw above, the vast majority of the molecules synthesized in a laboratory are comparatively small. By contrast, the medicaments obtained from microorganisms, animals, plants, or mushrooms — the so-called *biologics* — are much larger and generally less stable things, from molecules to cells, tissues, and whole organs. One of the most popular biologics is insulin, which nowadays is synthesized on an industrial scale by specially "trained" *Escherichia coli* bacteria. Also artemisin, the antimalarial drug, is being manufactured with the help of microorganisms — another triumph of synthetic biology, an emergent technology.

Other biologics of great interest to medicine are vaccines, mini-RNA, and monoclonal antibodies — in addition to blood, the oldest biologic. It is expected that biologics will become increasingly popular. Their development is using, and at the same time reinforcing, cell biology, bacteriology, and plant science — a reminder that any component of science is likely to help advance other components of it.

However, let us go back to synthetic chemistry. The starting point of a typical research project in this branch of pharmacology is a *lead molecule*. This is a compound that, in large quantities, possesses certain desirable physical and chemical properties, such as lipophilicity, or affinity with fats, and insolubility in water. (Lipophilicity is necessary to cross the cell membrane, which teems with lipids; and water solubility is necessary to move around in a medium that is basically watery.) Removing some atoms here, and adding or substituting others there, the lucky investigator will end up with a promising molecule: a *drug-like* one. (For a magisterial minitreatise on this subject, see Iversen 2001.)

For instance, if a drug is effective against a certain disease, but has adverse or just disagreeable side effects, the pharmacologist will attempt to design a similar molecule free from the said imperfections. For example, substituting a single H atom in the SO_2NH_2 molecule suffices to obtain a very different drug. Most of the psychoactive drugs currently prescribed by psychiatrists are comparatively small alterations of those introduced in the 1950s.

The preceding exemplifies the method of *successive approximations*, which is also the method of the sculptor who starts with a block of stone and, by successive chippings, transforms it into something that resembles more and more the image he has in mind. This procedure involves two important concepts that most philosophers have neglected: those of graded truth and efficacy.

The study of successive drug-like substances is not confined to their macrophysical properties; the diagram exhibiting the molecular structure of the drug-like substance also is looked at, to find out its similarities and differences with a known one. Every new molecule is subjected to trials, to discover whether, in fact, it is an effective and safe medical drug. These trials are so rigorous, that only about 4% of the drug-like substances pass it. Designing, testing, and marketing a new drug usually take several years of intense work and cost about two billion dollars — an estimated two-thirds of which go into marketing. This staggering cost has recently prompted a number of pharma firms to renege on the "Competition above all!" dogma of standard economic theory, and start working together to standardize drug trial formats.

Nor is it enough to pass a clinical trial; clinical experience may show, at the end of several years, the unforeseen imperfections of a drug. In fact, such experience may show not only that the drug has some nasty side effects, but also that its efficacy decreases with use ("tolerance"), or that it "interferes" with other drugs. For example, when taken in excess, Tylenol generates a toxic metabolite. (As soon as it is ingested or injected, a drug undergoes a whole sequence of chemical transformations, every phase of which is called a *metabolite*.)

As for tolerance, the prolonged consumption of a drug in large doses forces the liver to synthesize, in increasing quantities, the enzymes that degrade it, until that organ cannot keep up the race at the requisite pace, and the drug becomes ineffective. This is what happens with the nitrates employed to treat angina pectoris, or insufficient blood supply to the heart.

No one knows the suitable dose for natural remedies, because they are seldom put to rigorous trial. But of course, knowing the correct dose of a drug is just as important as knowing its pharmacodynamic properties, for an incorrect dose may be ineffective or fatal. (Even water will sicken or kill when ingested in excess, as any victim of the "enhanced interrogation technique" known as water-boarding will testify.) It has recently been conjectured that a high percentage of the victims of the Spanish influenza pandemic (1918–1920), which may have killed up to 100 million people, were poisoned by high doses of aspirin prescribed by the sanitary authorities. The underlying fallacy had been, of course, that the more of a good thing, the better.

To find out the desirable effects and the unanticipated side effects of a drug, in particular its possible toxicity above a certain dose, it is necessary to investigate the dose–response relation. Experiment has shown repeatedly that, in the vast majority of cases, a drug's effect first rises and then decreases with its concentration, until a point where a stronger cause ceases to translate into a stronger effect. (However, there is a large class of synthetic compounds, the so-called endocrine disruptors, that seem to provoke a stronger response at low levels — a counterintuitive result that has triggered an acrimonious controversy involving researchers, environmentalists, and the

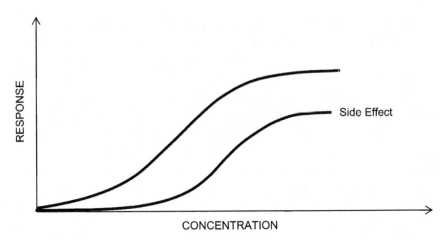

Fig. 5.1. The effect and side effect of a typical drug as a function of its dose. The curves are sigmoids.

drug industry.) This pattern, the "ski-slope" dose–response relation, illustrates the general principle that every causal relationship has a limited domain (Bunge 1959a). The optimal dose corresponds to the inflection point, beyond which adverse effects may occur — a reminder that in this field too there can be too much of a good thing. (See Figure 5.1.)

As suggested by the sigmoid curve, in typical cases, very small doses of anything, even of arsenic, are innocuous. Moreover, it is true that a glass of wine will "gladden the soul," as the Greeks say. (The mechanism is this: alcohol inhibits the brain inhibitors. This has initially a relaxing effect, which in turn eases socialization — the mechanism of parties.) Nevertheless, ethanol is a powerful toxic; it harms all of the organs, particularly the brain, and the typical adult can metabolize only 7–10 g (a small soup spoon) of alcohol per hour.

Besides, alcohol is addictive, which goes to explain the large percentage of alcoholism, a wrecker of personality and a severe social problem around the world. Therefore, it is irresponsible to keep repeating the wine industry's mantra: that wine is good for you when drunk in moderation. Wine is sold without warning, and the attempt to restrict its sale is a political hot potato, as the effect of prohibition and the fall of the Mendès France government remind us. But if preaching temperance is politically hazardous, affixing warning labels on wine bottles, as on cigarette packets, should eventually become as acceptable as sticking similar labels on cans of rat poison.

Sigmoid curves occur in all the sciences; they represent saturation processes with different mechanisms. At the chemical level, the saturation mechanism hinges on the valences of the atoms concerned. For example, the hydrogen atom cannot combine with more than one other hydrogen atom. The case of drug saturation in an organism is quite different; given that the amount of target enzyme is finite, there is no point in increasing the dose once the enzyme has finished the process of binding with it. The mechanism of the decline of epidemics is similar: they putter till they end, as the number of susceptible subjects decreases, by either immunization or death.

Finally, we must glance at *drug interaction*. For example, the mild and popular St. John's wort herb, a popular antidepressant sold without prescription, decreases the efficacy of oral contraceptives. Drug interaction is indirect: two or more drugs combine to form a harmful compound, but one of them competes with the other(s) for the enzyme that accelerates the metabolism of both. Such indirect competition is common at the chemical level; it is an instance of competition among processes — in this case, chemical reactions. The simplest case is that of competition of reactions of the forms $A + B \rightarrow C$ and $B + D \rightarrow E$, when they occur at the same place and time; both compete for the B reagent.

In sum, in the nations where medical drugs are controlled by the state, before putting them on the market, they have to be tried out, first in test tubes or Petri dishes, then in animals, and finally in hundreds or thousands of humans. Even so, it may happen that their shortcomings, such as serious side effects, appear only after they have been consumed by many thousands of subjects and have been the subject of many first-hand assays and meta-analyses. Thus, the drug consumer plays the role of an involuntary and unpaid guinea pig for the pharmaceutical industry.

When noticed, drug imperfections prompt both the pharmacologist and the industry to seek ever more effective and safer drugs. (This meritorious activity is called *pharmacovigilance*, but whistleblowers are seldom welcome.) Actually, imperfection has always motivated the innovator to do something to correct it. This is why it has been rightly said that science — unlike the market — is *self-corrective*. The same happens in technology too, but perhaps less often than in science because industrial retooling is so costly that it can hardly keep up with technological innovation. (Remember the time when big companies bought patents to prevent the manufacture of gadgets that would have driven their own outdated products out of the market?)

As noted above, pharmacologists try to design "clean" drugs that hit only specific targets (receptors). But sometimes, they churn out "dirty" drugs that affect multiple targets and consequently may have adverse effects. Still, occasionally, dirt pays, as was the case with chlorpromazine, first synthesized in 1950, and originally developed as a surgical anesthetic. The physician Henri Laborit noted that, besides alleviating pain, this drug has a remarkable calming effect, and in 1952 he used it successfully with psychotic patients. Two years later, Heinz Lehmann subjected the new drug to a rigorous and successful clinical trial, a result that consecrated it in the psychiatric community.

The success of this first antipsychotic was such that it revolutionized psychiatry, to the point that it led — prematurely, as it turned out — to closing down most of the insane asylums in the world. Chlorpromazine, the earliest successful psychoactive, was designed and used on the strength of a materialist philosophical hypothesis, namely psychoneural monism. It was also an unintended triumph of multiculturalism. In fact, Laborit, born in French Indochina, settled in Paris, and Lehmann was a German refugee who worked at McGill University, sited in the Anglophone enclave in Québec, the French America.

It was soon discovered, though, that chlorpromazine had some adverse effects, which motivated a sequence of redesigns. Still, the perfect antipsychotic remains elusive after six decades. Pharmacologists should not be blamed for this persistent imperfection; they cannot be expected to do better unless psychiatrists come up with a more precise diagnosis of schizophrenia, paranoia, and depression (recall Section 4.1). The moral is of course that pharmacology and the clinic should cooperate more closely for both to march in step.

In medicine, just as in basic science, every important new achievement leads to a new research line — by definition of 'important achievement.' In particular, the process of a pharmacological research project, from drug design to successful clinical trial to mass consumption, poses new problems at every step. Indeed, it defies the biochemist to make sure that the drug will be absorbed by the human gut; the chemical engineer to manufacture it on a large scale; the company manager to market it effectively; and the health professional to administer the drug in a tailor-made manner.

The passage from lab to market is called *translation* — a hot topic in the technology and business literatures. This complex process raises a number of issues, not only scientific and technological, but also moral and political, that lie beyond the borders of pharmacology. This is a disadvantage for the applied scientist and the technologist relative to the basic scientist: that, because they need to court economic and political powers, they may get entangled in disputes and manoeuvers that have to do more with the ownership of truth than with the search for it.

5.3 Philosophical Dividends

Dialectics and reductionism are two of the most popular philosophical ideas among scientists. Dialectics, though invented by Hegel, is best known to scientists in Friedrich Engels' (1883) version, and reductionism is widely believed to be the ultimate goal of science. Hence, both doctrines deserve being analyzed.

The center of dialectical ontology is the opaque postulate of the "struggle and unity of opposites": every thing would be a "unity of opposites"; every change would result from some conflict; and every qualitatively new stage in a process would "negate" the preceding one. Assuming charitably that the concepts of dialectical opposition and negation were unproblematic, a few counterexamples should suffice to confute the given thesis.

The building blocks of the universe, such as electrons and photons, are simple, and yet always in flux; cooperation coexists with conflict and even trumps the latter because it generates systems; and every entity is either a system or a system component. In particular, every human being is a system composed of subsystems, such as the cardiovascular and the nervous ones, every one of which is in turn composed of subsystems, such as organs, down to the cellular level and further down. Moreover, any conflict within or between such systems, as when a limb fails to obey the brain, is a dysfunction that demands medical assistance. In sum, to the extent that it is intelligible, dialectics is false — except for its emphasis on change.

As for reductionism, it may be radical or moderate. The four (or five) elements and the humoral doctrines we met in the first chapter were radically reductionist. So is the contemporary opinion that an organism is nothing but a batch of molecules. Ditto the geneticism advanced by Richard Dawkins, who holds that organisms are nothing but funnels for transmitting inalterable genes from one generation to the next, so that their very existence is paradoxical. This, the most modern and fashionable version of nativism, was recently refuted by the discovery of epigenetics, the chapter of genetics that deals with methylation and other inheritable chemical alterations of genes as a consequence of the organism's interactions with its environment. Actually, the nature/nurture dilemma had been resolved decades earlier, both in biology and in psychology, in favor of a combination of nature with nurture. The individualism inherent in contemporary social science is no better, as it fails to explain why people struggle to get into or out of social systems, from families to business firms to political parties. The very idea of a social science without social systems is an oxymoron.

All of these versions of radical reductionism are false because they overlook or even deny *emergence*: the fact that systems have global properties, such as life, age, developmental stage, and life history, that their parts lack. The recognition of emergence goes together with the invention of the corresponding ideas, such as those of development and evolution, metabolism, and immunity. That is also why every level of organization has its peculiar patterns or laws, which is why the fractals fad — based on the similarity of things at all levels — has been barren.

For the same reason, biology is not applied chemistry, nor is chemistry the boring part of physics, as physicists used to think. What is true is that the *constituents* of the things on the nth level of organization belong in level $n-1$. And, whereas the former are studied by science S_n, their next-level constituents are studied by science S_{n-1}. Thus, physics and chemistry precede biology because they study cell components, and in turn biology precedes social science because human groups are ultimately composed of persons. That is, the *epistemological* precedence relation is rooted in the *ontological* part–whole relation (Bunge 1969, 1979, 2004; Anderson 1972). This example suggests that the theory of knowledge cannot get very far without a theory of being and becoming, or ontology, and it explains why the former has not helped account for the "hierarchy" of the sciences. Back to reductionism, the research strategy that attempts to transform every discipline into a lower-level one.

The strong point of vitalism, in its centuries-long battle with physical and physico-chemical reductionism, was that it emphasized the peculiarities of organisms, such as their autonomy, resilience, and self-repairing ability. However, admitting these characteristics does not commit one to the fuzzy notions of entelechy (Aristotle) and *élan vital* (Bergson), since self-organization processes occur at several levels in addition to the biotic one; witness the spontaneous formation of snow crystals out of atmospheric moisture, and the birth of informal or spontaneous human associations.

To admit emergence without miracle, it suffices to adopt the systemic conception first articulated by d'Holbach (1770, 1773), whom we met in Chapter 2. Indeed, according to systemism, every concrete thing is either a system or an actual or potential constituent of a system; every system has properties that its constituents lack; and systems are grouped into levels of organization (Bunge 1979). In sum, *systemism implies emergentism*, and in principle every case of emergence can be accounted for in scientific terms, instead of having to be accepted as a miracle. To be sure, both hypotheses, systemism and emergentism, are philosophical, since they transcend disciplinary borders, but they are not extravagant speculations, since they are supported by contemporary science, which is neither physicalist (downward reduction) nor spiritualist (upward reduction).

Systemism is tacitly adopted every time the object of study is treated as a complex and cohesive thing with global properties as well as interacting with its environment. However, systemism is rarely embraced in an explicit fashion, and it is often confused with other doctrines. The most common confusions are its equation with holism, and the idea that systematization rigidifies. The first confusion dissipates upon recalling that holism opposes analysis, whereas systemism suggests analyzing every concrete system into its composition, environment, structure, and mechanism (recall Section 2.3).

As for the second confusion, it may be due to the fact that the best-known conceptual systems are the theologies and the ossified philosophies — all of which claim to have solved all problems once and for all. This is why the phrase *esprit de système* is often used in a derogatory manner. But the systemism practiced in the sciences is not static, and it does not conceive of all systems as closed and in equilibrium. (Talcott Parson's sociology, whose influence peaked in the 1950s, is the outstanding exception.) In particular, all biologists and physicians take it for granted that human beings are open systems in a state of flux.

Since humans cross all the levels of organization, from the atomic to the social, they cannot be understood or managed if flattened to a single level. In particular, the common cold is an infection caused by the rhinovirus which affects our intellect and social life, and cancer begins with a DNA mutation and alters the cancerous person's social behavior; by contrast, stress starts at the social level and goes down to the molecular level, for it stimulates the synthesis of corticoids, which in turn harm tissues.

Moderate reduction is welcome for reminding us that we are multilevel systems, so that we must be studied at all levels, as well as that, whereas some processes remain on a given level, others move from the bottom up, and still others from the top down. Hence, we must admit processes of three kinds, both in reality and in its exploration: same-level, bottom-up, and top-down. Pharmacologists adopt all three, which helps explain their spectacular successes in the course of the last hundred years. Suffice it to recall the following firsts: antibiotics (1933), antipsychotics (1952), antidepressants (1955), oral contraceptives (1960), antihypertensives (1962), anticholesterols (1985), plus a number of vaccines that have saved uncounted children, from the triple vaccine to the first effective and safe vaccine to prevent gastroenteritis (2006).

As noted above, before 1900, effective medical intervention was confined to surgery and a few medicaments extracted from plants — some of which, alas, turned out to be toxic. Nowadays, there are far less invasive surgical procedures, as well as hundreds of effective synthetic drugs. Even clinical psychology and psychiatry are quickly going from shamanism to protoscience. Every single branch of medicine has been updated in light of biomedical research. Yet, many bureaucrats and statesmen have still to learn that biomedical research languishes unless basic science prospers at the same time.

In general, when adapted to medicine, engineering, or politics, a basic science gets transformed into an applied science. And in turn, an applied science is "translated" into a technology when it guides the design of artifacts, such as medical drugs, therapies, machines, nursing practices, and public health policies. Since about 1800, a good medical school has hosted basic scientists (in particular anatomists, physiologists, and cellular biologists);

applied scientists (in particular pharmacologists and clinical psychologists); technologists (in particular prostheses and therapeutics designers); and craftsmen (in particular nurses and hospital administrators).

There are two information flows between these fields: the transmission of findings and that of problems.

Knowledge

$\rightarrow$

Basic science   Applied science   Technology   Craft

$\leftarrow$

Problems

Coda

The traditional Chinese pharmacopeia consists of about 12,000 natural products, and the Ayurvedic of more than 7,000 compounds derived from plants. But nobody knows the composition of any of those alleged remedies, and it is known that only a few of them are mildly effective, others just placebos, and still others harmful. The scientific pharmacopeia is far more reduced, and the composition and medical effects of every member of it are fairly well known; in some cases the mechanism of action is known as well. All this is due to their being found or made and tested scientifically, and to the fact that their sales are subject to two supreme rules: safety and effectiveness proved by rigorous clinical trials — not by authority or hearsay.

Still, spontaneous ignorance and the myths invented by charlatans and postmodern scribblers are such that shamans are still listened to, particularly in the so-called developing regions. Most of the people in those regions cannot afford remedies made to the measure of far deeper pockets. The net result is that there are two pharmacopeias: the effective one for the rich and the ineffective one for the poor. For better or for worse, pharmacologists can do nothing to solve this social problem.

Philosophers ought to help design conceptual filters to separate pseudo-remedies from genuine medicaments. But few, if any, philosophers have collaborated in this task. Most of them are more interested in conceptual or verbal games than in real-world problems, such as that of health. Worse, some of them, from Hegel and Nietzsche to Husserl and Heidegger, to Foucault and Derrida, have attacked the scientific endeavor; or, like

Wittgenstein, Kripke, and David Lewis, they have escaped both the real world and its investigation. If you wish effective medication, support scientific investigation (see Bunge 2012a). And if you wish investigation, cultivate a philosophy that may help it.

Let us next glance at the assay of drugs, required by both scientificity and morals.

Chapter 6

TRIAL

6.1 Clinical Trial

Therapies, like songs, are invented. But, unlike a song, a therapy is neither adopted nor discarded on the strength of taste or opinion. The primitive healers applied therapies backed by tradition and accompanied by magical or religious rituals. The Hippocratic and Galenic medics discarded magic and religion, and trusted experience and the four-humors doctrine. Besides, their therapy was sober: bed rest, light meals, and barley water. It was only in later centuries that bloodletting became the panacea and consequently was overused. In any event, the Hippocratic and Galenic treatments relied on *some* evidence, albeit some of it imaginary — just like the procedures of the engineer and the judge, neither of which was either arbitrary or perfect.

The design of scientific therapies is far more demanding; besides passing rigorous clinical trials, they must be plausible in light of extant knowledge. (For a different take, see Howick 2011.) The *plausibility* or *verisimilitude* of a therapy consists in its compatibility with the bulk of biomedical knowledge, and it is assessed prior to any trials. For example, homeopathy is utterly implausible if only because the homeopathic preparations are so highly diluted that they are unlikely to contain even one molecule of the alleged active principle. By contrast, it is possible that an antiviral drug designed to disable or even destroy virions of a specific kind will be effective to treat the disease caused by them.

Note two points. First, before the rise of medicine proper, it was usual to demand of a therapy that it should be consistent with the prevailing prescientific worldview. Second, one should demand compatibility with the *bulk*, not the totality of the background knowledge, because the latter

129

is bound to contain falsehoods. The importance of new rigorous trials increases when the compatibility condition is not met.

In modern medicine, clinical trials are expected to be rigorous; they cannot be confined to a handful of clinical cases without controls, that is, mere anecdotes. Sometimes tests of this kind demote old "proven" remedies that had been used on the sole basis of experience, not experiment. A recent casualty is cod liver oil supplement, widely used for more than a century to prevent a number of diseases; a meta-analysis conducted on 68,000 subjects (Rizos *et al.* 2012) found that it is neither good nor bad for the heart. Incidentally, the mechanism of action of the said health supplement has never been clear (more on this in the Coda).

A therapy can be said to be *scientifically plausible*, or *well founded*, just in case its mechanism of action is known or suspected with some biological ground. For example, if simulations *in vitro* or *in silico* show that a certain drug blocks the production of virions of some kind, it is considered as a plausible candidate to treat the corresponding viral infection. In this case, the researcher conducts a preclinical trial on animal "models" before trying it on human guinea pigs. Such trials presuppose that humans, though very special, are animals after all, so that what works for cancerous rats may also work for cancerous humans.

If no possible mechanism of action for a therapy exists, its further study won't be worthwhile. This is the case of the magico-religious therapies, as well as of acupuncture and homeopathy, all of which act at most as placebos (see Section 7.2). In particular, it should be obvious that those therapies can do nothing about diseases with a cellular root, such as diabetes, and even less about those with a molecular root, such as cancer.

How do we know that a medical treatment is effective? The vulgar answer is: because it helped some people. But how many or, better, in what percentage? This question was not even asked until 1835, when Pierre Louis put in practice his *méthode numérique* to check the effectiveness of bloodletting to treat pneumonia. He found what the contemporary reader might expect: that bloodletting did not help.

From then on, biomedical researchers have looked for success percentages as well as for possible side effects. That is, they wish to know not only whether a treatment is effective, but also whether it is *efficient* (high output/input ratio). For instance, until 2011, the treatments for hepatitis C — which can remain asymptomatic for decades — were quite effective but had also serious side effects, as they did not dismantle the virus but only prevented it from multiplying. This suggests looking not only for results, but also for mechanisms of action (more on this further down).

Personal experience, however rich, is untransferable, and often ineffable as well. And, being subjective, it lacks scientific value, although it may motivate scientific research. Besides, personal experience is confined to the perceptible; it does not include imperceptible things like enzymes and viruses, or imperceptible processes such as loss of bone density and hemolysis. For these reasons, researchers in the sciences and technologies dealing with the real world conduct experiments; these alone, along with controlled speculation, can ferret out and manipulate the unseen.

Medical schools teach one to observe and measure, but only rarely to design and execute experiments. In contradistinction to an observation, an experiment consists in *wiggling suspect variables* to discover the effects, if any, of such variation. In other words, as Claude Bernard (1865) explained, *an experiment is an intervention explained, designed and controlled in light of some causal hypothesis.* Note that the entire sentence in italics is philosophical as well as scientific — as befits a piece of methodology, or normative epistemology.

Let us insist on the importance of hypotheses in scientific experiment. The most common hypotheses in biomedical research are (a) the *null hypothesis* (that two or more given variables are not associated); (b) *general alternative hypotheses* of the forms "X is a cause of that disease," "The course of that disease is such and such," "The mechanism of X is Y," and "This therapy may help treat that disorder"; and (c) *particular hypotheses*, of the forms "This individual is likely to suffer from that disease," "This individual qualifies for that therapy," and "This protocol is likely to help that patient."

The aim of an experiment, contrary to that of an observation or a measurement, is to garner empirical data relevant to a hypothesis, to test it and find out its *degree of factual* (or *empirical*) *truth* (true, true within such an error, or false). When there is a theory (hypothetico-deductive system of propositions) referring to the same facts, the hypothesis that undergoes an empirical test can also be assigned a *theoretical truth value*. In both cases, the truth in question is factual, not formal or mathematical. That is, what one seeks in factual science and medicine are hypotheses fitting the facts they refer to and, if possible, also supported by previously found hypotheses.

(The capital distinction between *truths of fact* and *truths of reason* was clearly drawn by Leibniz nearly four centuries ago, but it is still being ignored by most logicians and philosophers. The main reasons for upholding the factual/formal distinction are that factual truths refer to facts and are checked by empirical means, such as observation and experiment, whereas formal truths do not refer to facts and are checked by purely conceptual means. An additional reason is that all of the logical statements, and most of the mathematical ones, are fully true, whereas the sciences and technologies produce mostly *approximately* true propositions. See Bunge 1974b.)

In contemporary physics and chemistry, hypotheses are not subject to costly experimental tests unless they are compatible with reasonably well-established theories. Heterodoxies are welcome as long as they do not violate the most basic laws. True, some cosmologists speculate about the creation of the universe out of nothing, or even about the coexistence of many mutually disconnected universes, but these unscientific fantasies are seldom taken seriously because they do not connect with any empirical data.

Even in the biomedical sciences, so poor in theories, heterodox hypotheses are expected to comply with the bulk of biomedical science before they are considered for experimental tests. For instance, not even a religious scientist would design a trial to test the hypothesis that walking to Lourdes will cure cancer.

In all the sciences, regardless of their level of development, negative or confuting data are just as appreciated as positive or corroborating ones. The weight assigned to an empirical datum relevant to a given hypothesis depends on the latter's theoretical status. If it is an isolated or free-standing hypothesis, that is, one lacking theoretical support — as is the case with all the empirical generalizations — then it is reasonable to assign a greater value to the negative data than to the positive ones. The reason for this rule is purely logical: because the inference "If A, then B. Now, not-B. Hence, not-A" is conclusive (valid), whereas "If A, then B. Now, B. Hence A," is fallacious (invalid). In other words, in the immature sciences, it is advisable to adopt the *refutationist* strategy recommended by Popper (1935), in opposition to the *confirmationism* or *inductivism* preached by the positivists such as Rudolf Carnap, Hans Reichenbach, and at one time Bertrand Russell as well.

But in the mature sciences, negative data are not more valuable than the positive ones; much depends on the track record of the hypothesis in question. For example, in 2011, a team of Italian physicists announced that they had found neutrinos traveling faster than light in a vacuum. If this were true, then the special theory of relativity would be false. But this theory is deeply embedded in physics, and it has been confirmed by myriad measurements in the course of one century, hence the alleged negative result must have involved an experimental error. This is why few physicists believe the said result, which was soon withdrawn.

In short, refutationism only holds for isolated hypotheses. In the mature sciences, theoretical truth may trump any number of isolated negative data (Bunge 1967). This explains why crucial experiments — those that allow one to make clear choices among competing hypotheses — are far less frequent in the mature sciences than in the underdeveloped ones (Bunge 1968, 1973).

Every time a research project in the biomedical sciences is evaluated by a granting agency, the first point to be considered is its *biological plausibility*, or consistency with the relevant background knowledge. For example, a project designed to test whether humans can live without oxygen, or would not get sick if injected syphilis bacilli, would be discarded without further ado. It is wrong for philosophers of science to keep analyzing isolated hypotheses, because modern science is a system; only protoscience and pseudoscience are collections of unrelated or weakly related beliefs. However, back to experimental design.

It is well known that every biomedical experiment involves two groups of organisms: the experimental and the control. The former is constituted by the individuals that will receive the stimulus, whereas the control (or witness) group is composed by the ones that won't get it. For example, on noting that boiling oil did not heal shot wounds, Paracelsus (1536) tried a salve that turned out to be more effective — or at least less harmful — than the traditional treatment. He proceeded by trial and error, without the guide of guesses on possible mechanisms of action. His only hypothesis was that maybe the salve was more effective than boiling oil because at least it did not fry the flesh. But Paracelsus did not confine himself to counting favorable cases; he split his group of wounded soldiers into two groups, the way the experimental method requires, and noted the difference in healing times.

Since Claude Bernard's path-breaking experiments on glycogen (1857) — the sugar-forming substance in the liver — biomedical researchers have not groped in the dark, but have been guided by hypotheses. Most of these are not arbitrary fantasies but, as noted above, educated guesses, that is, conjectures compatible with the bulk of biomedicine. Paracelsus had been unable to proceed in this way, because the medicine of his time was protoscientific; in particular, it knew nothing about mechanisms of action. Bernard, by contrast, could use the chemistry, cellular biology, and physiology that had been learned in the course of the three preceding centuries; he could, and did, think up some *scientific* hypotheses, so intriguing that they sparked off memorable experiments, like the one that produced rabbits with floppy ears.

Bernard's experiments were not haphazard trials, like those of the professor of medicine who forced his lab animals to swallow cleaning products of unknown composition, just to see what happened to them. Ditto the pseudo-experiments conducted by the Nazi doctors on inmates of concentration camps; none of them produced new knowledge, because they were not designed to test any scientific hypotheses and did not involve controls; they were like the trials that untutored children perform with their first chemistry sets.

The unique virtue of the scientific experiment is not that it yields new data, but that it combines extant data with plausible hypotheses, and involves the control of variables of possible interest. A *scientific hypothesis*, such as the one on the combination of hemoglobin with oxygen, or on the action of a drug on a receptor, is both (a) empirically testable and (b) compatible with the bulk of the relevant background knowledge.

Moreover, an experiment may, and often does, refer to facts that are inaccessible to direct observation, whence the futility of inductive logic (Bunge 2012a). For this reason, a scientific hypothesis cannot be put to the test without the aid of *indicators* or *markers*, in particular biomarkers bridging the observed facts with the ones, usually on other levels, that cannot be observed in a direct manner. For example, pulse rate is an indicator of cardiac pumping, and high body temperature usually indicates infection.

For the same reason, scientific hypotheses cannot be contrasted directly with data, but have to be conjoined with indicators — or, as it used to be said, they have to be "operationalized." For example,

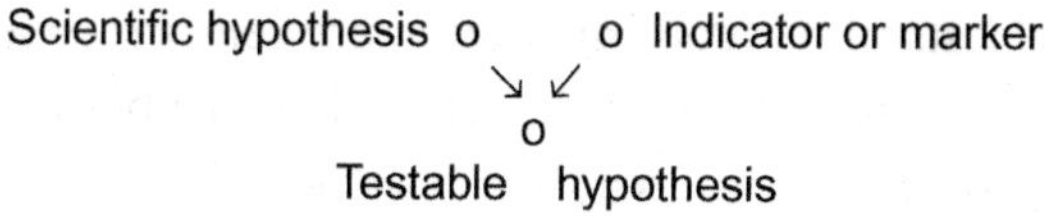

Scientific hypothesis o   o Indicator or marker

            ↘ ↙

           o

Testable   hypothesis

Fig. 6.1. Translation of a scientific hypothesis into empirical terms by means of an indicator hypothesis (from Bunge 1967, Vol. 2).

a hypothesis involving the temperature concept will have to be conjoined with a temperature–thermometer reading indicator. In other words, to put a theoretical hypothesis to the experimental test, it is necessary to translate it into observable signs, such as pointer readings (see Figure 6.1).

Any experimental investigator knows the differences between experiment and observation. The best-known difference between them is that an experiment involves the comparison of two groups of things: the experimental and the control (or witness). This is done to find out the effect of a stimulus, as when the members of the former group are given a drug that is not given to those in the control group (more on this in Section 6.2).

Let us now comment on a less well-known peculiarity of experiment and, indeed, of precision measurement as well. Experimental designs involve the use or invention of *indicators* (or *markers*) that disclose some traits of imperceptible things, processes, or properties. In other words, the measurement and experimental control of an imperceptible variable V, such as body temperature, is done through some marker M that maps V. Thus, when reading a classical mercury clinical thermometer, we read the mercury level on a scale that translates centimeters into degrees Celsius via the physical law "$L = L_0(1 + \alpha t)$", where L_0 stands for length at temperature $t = 0$. Something similar happens with all the other properties that cannot be accessed directly with the unaided senses. (More on indicators in Bunge 1967, 2012a.)

Although indicators are ubiquitous in experimental science, none of the better-known philosophers of science, whether inductivists like Carnap or refutationists like Popper, deal with them when discussing measurement or experiment; they presuppose that all hypotheses are confronted directly with the relevant empirical evidence. Hence, all their writings about testability, confirmation, and refutation sound hollow. Ian Hacking (1983) did not mention them either in a book that made him famous overnight because it revealed that scientists intervene actively besides observing passively — something that Francis Bacon had stressed more than three centuries earlier. Nor did Bas van Fraassen (2008) in a much-cited book where he held that general theories yield experimental data. Actually, all experiments and all precision measurements call for their own specific indicators.

(Yet, it is a dogma of the standard or Copenhagen interpretation of quantum mechanics that "every eigenvalue [of an operator representing a dynamical variable] is the possible result of the measurement of the dynamical variable for some state of the system" [Dirac 1958: 36]. But this is false. For example, there is no instrument to measure the energy values calculated by means of the theory; a spectrograph, in combination with a comparator, yields only light frequencies, which atomic theory converts into energy differences.)

Every science that studies a bit of reality involves either experiments or theories in other fields that have passed experimental trials. The traumatologist, who claims that his craft requires no experiment because all he needs to know and do is in clear view, should be informed that, if responsible, he will not improvise like Madame Bovary's pathetic husband. The philosopher who objects that astronomers do not experiment should be told that astronomy employs theories, like those of mechanics, gravitation, and optics, that have passed stringent laboratory tests. Likewise, those who claim that it is impossible to make social experiments are to be informed that social experiments have been made for over a century.

Let us briefly recall one of the most famous social experiments: the Hawthorne Study (1924–1932) in an American utilities firm. The underlying hypothesis was that labor productivity would increase if management showed that it cared for its personnel. The lighting was improved, the walls were repainted in bright colors, and a cafeteria was installed. Productivity rose as predicted, and since then there has been plenty of talk of the "Hawthorne effect." But since there were no control groups, no experiment proper was conducted. Moreover, a study published six decades later (Jones 1992) showed that the researchers had missed the Great Depression (1929–1939), which started in the middle of the "experiment." And this factor suffices to explain the rise in productivity: the employees worked harder for fear of losing their jobs. The *post hoc, ergo propter hoc* fallacy had been committed. Still, the Hawthorne Study had unwittingly corroborated another hypothesis: that economic insecurity keeps workers on their toes.

The only experimental attempt ever made by psychoanalysts in the course of one century (Vaughan *et al.* 2000) ignored the essential requirement of the experimental method: it did not include a control group. The first correct evaluation of a psychoanalytic treatment was made one decade later (Sørensen *et al.* 2011), and concluded that the improvement was undistinguishable from a placebo effect. So, psychoanalysis has been practiced for more than a century without a shred of evidence of its effectiveness. Doctor Placebo has been in attendance without collecting the fees charged by the analysts.

Medical experiments can be of either the laboratory or the clinical type. In the former case, they are conducted to find *truths* as to what causes specific diseases and what alters their courses. By contrast, clinical trials are done to find out the *effectiveness* of the various proposed therapies. (But, of course, an effectiveness trial seeks to determine whether or not it is *true* that a certain therapy works. There is no escaping the concept of truth.) The motivations for trials of both types are curiosity, peer recognition, and possible utility. The basic scientist, by contrast, is motivated only by curiosity and peer recognition (Merton 1973).

Medical trials are conducted on several levels. For example, if what is being tried is a drug, it will be applied to cells in a test tube, to tissues in a Petri dish, to organs immersed in a saline solution, or to whole animals. All these levels have to be investigated, not only to find out the effectiveness of the drug, but also to determine the *therapeutic window*, that is, the interval of maximal effectiveness. This requires tracing the dose–response curve, as discussed in Section 5.2. Interestingly, the said therapeutic window matches a *moral window*. This is the Hippocratic and Stoic rule of moderation: nothing good serves in tiny doses, and it may turn out to be harmful when used in excess. Thus, one of the virtues of scientific medicine is that, because it adopts a scientistic strategy and a humanist ethics, it seeks the coincidence of the therapeutic and moral windows.

However, in some cases, the said moral window is so narrow as to be useless; this happens with treatments for conditions so severe that it is impractical or immoral to use placebo-controlled groups. Progeria is a case in point. This is a rare genetic disease characterized by very rapid aging and severe complications, such as stroke. Its victims die on average at age 12, looking 90. Who would have the heart to try a new promising drug on only some of them while giving placebos to the others? By the time the trial was over, no subjects might survive.

Another philosophical aspect of biomedical experimentation is that, although contemporary biomedical research may start at the molecular level, it cannot stay in it. This is because organelles, cells, and organs have global (emergent) properties, such as apoptosis (programmed death) in the case of cells, and blood pressure in that of cardiovascular systems. Thus, to understand whether a hypertensive drug works, it must be tried on whole animals; but to understand how it works (i.e., its mechanism), it will be necessary to go down several steps.

Let us close this section by warning against the fashionable idea that "facts are theory laden." That it is absurd is shown by well-known facts such as that the obesity epidemic started long before epidemiologists took notice of it. Only the *data sought in the advanced sciences* can be theory laden, in that they are produced with the help of procedures, such as the MRI, that make sense only in light of hypotheses subject to correction. Health policies, too, are theory laden. But the effects of the application of such policies, such as changes in morbidity and mortality rates, are just as real as the oceans.

6.2 Chance Can Help Find Causes

The main goal of clinical studies is to measure the "effect size" of the treatment that is being studied. The studies in question can be primary, or bearing on people, or secondary. The latter, called *meta-analyses*, are studies of primary studies. In the terminology advocated by the Cochrane Collaboration (2013), a meta-analysis is "the use of statistical techniques in a systematic review to integrate the results of included studies." Note the word *results*, of which more in Section 6.3.

Such a measurement — or rather estimation — of the size of the effect of a medical treatment is not attained in purely observational studies, where health states before and after the treatment are compared. Claude Bernard

(1865) argued eloquently that it is not enough to check what happens after the stimulus has been applied; it is also necessary to see how the organism behaves when the stimulus is *not* applied. In other words, two groups of organisms of the same species and in similar states must be studied: the experimental and the control (or witness). The members of the former, or *experimental group E*, are treated, whereas the ones in the *control group C*, are not.

Without controls, one risks committing the *post hoc, ergo propter hoc* fallacy ("after that, hence because of that"). This is a fallacy because the change in health state may be due to a different cause, such as self-suggestion or mood improvement, either of which may alter the immune reaction through some psycho-neuro-endocrine chain triggered by the patient's belief in the treatment. (More on placebo effects in Section 7.2.) We shall call the *silver standard* (by analogy with the gold standard) the rule that Bernard first articulated and practiced consistently.

The adoption of the silver standard in biomedical research was crucial, but not the final word. Indeed, starting in 1948, clinical trials were expected to be even more rigorous; they involve not only control groups, but also *randomization*, that is, the random choice of the members of the experimental and control groups. That year, the team led by Geoffrey Marshall, at the British Medical Research Council, concluded the first *randomized, placebo-controlled, and double-blind* clinical trial. That trial, designed by the biostatistician Austin Bradford Hill, proved the efficacy of the recently invented streptomycin to cure pulmonary tuberculosis in humans. (Note the word *proved*, proscribed by empiricism long ago.) Methodological rigor yielded an unexpected sensational result: millions of persons around the world were cured in a short time from one of the most serious and refractory diseases. (See Figure 6.2.)

Randomization is expected to guarantee that the experimental and control groups be initially *equivalent* on average, that is, free from involuntary bias. In other words, randomization prevents the researcher from inadvertently influencing the choice of subjects so as to maximize the chance of success of his pet hypothesis. (Remember the proverbial if imaginary case of the doctor who tried an anti-seasick pill only on his ship's crew, so as not to inconvenience the passengers.)

The ideas of random choice and random trial had been used in experimental agriculture two decades earlier by Ronald Fisher (1935), eminent

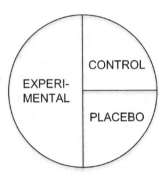

Fig. 6.2. The experimental subjects are allotted at random to two groups: the experimental group, whose members are given the therapy under test, and the rest, or control group. The latter, in turn, is split into two: those who are not given anything, and those who are given a dummy treatment or placebo.

statistician, geneticist, agronomist, evolutionary biologist — and eugenicist. The crux of a randomized trial, whether in agriculture, industry, or medicine, is the formation of the E and C groups. The allotment of individuals to each of these two groups is random, or double-blind, as well as placebo-controlled if possible. Chance may be generated by tossing a coin, using a random-numbers table, or some other method.

The members of the two groups are examined periodically and, at the end of the trial, the experimenter notes the differences, if any, between the treated individuals and the witnesses. The end result is judged to be favorable to the therapy in question if it passes a *statistical significance* test. There are several tests of this kind. The most popular of them is the χ^2, or chi-squared, which involves a measure of the differences in the values of the trait that is being investigated.

The formation of experimental and control groups is a matter of routine everywhere but in medicine, where it is delicate and expensive, as well as annoying or even harmful to the subjects. Think of the clinical trials of promising new drugs on humans — mostly young males. The professional guinea pigs are typically destitute individuals in poor health, therefore susceptible to comorbidities, which complicates the task of finding the specific effects of the drug in question.

Because of its impartiality, it has been agreed almost universally that a medical treatment is effective if and only if it has passed *randomized clinical trials* or RCTs (Bradford Hill 1937). This has been called the *gold standard* of experimental medicine. This denomination is a *convention* or agreement, not a law of nature. So much so, that there are still dissidents, not only in the medical community, but also in the pharmaceutical industry, which has complained about the slowness and high cost of such trials.

The critics of RCTs forget that too many failed therapies have been used on the sole basis of "observational studies." For example, the hormonal replacement therapy used over more than two decades to prevent heart diseases in postmenopausal women, turned out to *increase* the risk of coronary heart disease when subjected to an RCT. This historic trial involved 16,000 women observed over half a dozen years, and its results were published in 2012, more than half a century after the first successful RCT (Andreoli *et al.* 2010: 743). Nobody knows how many lives were lost by (a) the refusal to adopt the gold standard, and (b) the extraordinary belief that menopause is a disease, and such a serious one that it warrants messing with women's endocrine systems.

A common objection to the RCT is that physicists and chemists obtain far more precise data without randomizing. This is true, but there are good reasons for this exception. First, physicists and chemists can use potent searchlights that are not available to physicians, namely general and well-confirmed theories involving key variables, and sometimes mechanisms of action as well. Second, in the so-called "hard" sciences, the experimenter can wiggle and measure, albeit indirectly in most cases, all the key variables, which is seldom the case in the other disciplines because such variables are rarely known, precisely because of the dearth of medical theories.

Third, physicists and chemist can handle *homogeneous* populations, constituted by entities of the same species. By contrast, the biomedical and social researchers work typically on *heterogeneous* populations, that is, collections of individuals of different origins and with different life histories. Surely, their members share many traits — for example, they are all diabetic adolescents with a sedentary lifestyle — but they differ among one another in all remaining respects, most of them unknown or deliberately ignored in order to find general patterns.

Such heterogeneity makes it necessary to choose at random the subjects of a study, so that the unknown variables will be equally represented in the experimental and the control groups. This alone will guarantee that both groups are as *equivalent* as possible, so that the intervention stands out as the *only cause* of the difference in the outcome of the study. A similar consideration — avoidance of privilege — led the ancient Athenians to appoint their magistrates by lots. Randomization is egalitarian.

(The heterogeneity of populations of organisms is usually called *variability*, but actually what is meant is *variety* or *diversity*. Variation, a process that takes time, may cause diversity and therefore heterogeneity, but the converse is not always true. The degree of variety in a given variable or property is measured by its *variance*, a statistical parameter that is just as important as the *mode* or *median*. In the particular but frequent case of a bell-shaped distribution, the variance is the average bell width.)

Most RCTs yield net results. When they don't, the experimental result is revised and a new trial is conducted. Even so, the outcome may not be conclusive; it may only be a "definite maybe." Whether or not the outcome is decisive, if promising, the trial deserves being supplemented by investigating the next question: why might the therapy in question be effective? In other words, which are the *mechanisms of action* of both pathogenesis and treatment? The drug used to prevent esophageal cramps acts as a muscle relaxant; oral contraceptives stop ovulation; and streptomycin kills the Koch bacillus by inhibiting its protein synthesis — a molecular process so complex that it is still being investigated.

The case of streptomycin to treat pulmonary tuberculosis should draw the philosopher's attention for several reasons. First, although that disease has obvious symptoms, such as low fever, coughing, and bloody sputum, its treatment with an antibiotic starts at the molecular level but has social repercussions, such as contagion, isolation, reinsertion in society — and the erstwhile lucrative sanatoria industry. In short, the process goes through several levels of organization. Consequently, knowing the molecular process in question — the mutation that inhibits protein synthesis in the pathogen — is not sufficient to understand the patient's recovery; all the relevant levels must be taken into consideration. Something similar holds for mental disorders; although they happen inside the patient's skull, they have social repercussions because the brain connects the person with her environment. However, back to the general features of the randomized trial.

The most fecund trials are those that, on top of solving an important problem, raise further questions. For example, although acupuncture has been practiced on billions of persons over more than two millennia, it has never inspired any fruitful biomedical research projects, and it was subjected to experimental tests only recently. One of the most interesting trials was the one conducted by Daniel C. Cherkin and 12 coworkers (2009). A group of 638 individuals suffering from chronic lumbar pain was divided into two subgroups: the experimental and the control. In turn, the former was split into three: (a) those who were pricked with standard needles at the places indicated by the traditional anatomical drawings, drawn 1,500 years before the birth of anatomy; (b) the ones who were pricked at random with standard needles; and (c) those who received sham acupuncture with toothpicks. The members of the control group received the standard treatment: bed rest.

What is surprising is not that sham acupuncture gave the same result as the traditional one, but that all the pricked subjects felt a notable improvement relative to the controls. The researchers concluded that they do not know whether the improvement is a placebo effect or an unknown physiological process that raises the pain threshold. Presumably, if the pain mechanisms were better known, it might be possible to design a *nocimeter* to measure objectively pain intensities, and the same instrument could be used to experiment on animals impervious to beliefs.

In sum, only RCTs allow researchers to find out whether a medical treatment is effective. (If preferred, this method is used to find out whether propositions of the form "This therapy is effective" are true or false.) Still, the results obtained through that method need not be definitive; different trials may conflict with one another either because of flaws in design or because adverse or side effects may mask the central process. But more research can resolve such conflicts.

Therapies and trial designs can be improved or discarded; scientific medicine is imperfect but perfectible, whereas the medical sects are unchangeable. Hence, the psychological difference between the adherent to scientific medicine and the uncritical believer in a CAM: whereas the former trusts the research process, the sectarian keeps faith with a finished product. And, since he trusts neither research results nor debates with skeptics, controversies with him tend to be acrimonious and unending, unless the believer terminates them stating, "But it worked for me, and that is enough for me."

6.3 Methodological Controversies

The convention that the RCT is the *gold standard* of scientific medicine has been criticized often and from its inception. One of the most influential criticisms is that it has not produced any scientific discoveries (Rubin 1974). This claim is true, but it misses the point of the said trials, which is not to generate new medical ideas, but to evaluate interventions on heterogeneous populations.

Another much-cited opinion is that of Hayward and Krumholz (2012): "The critical component of good clinical decision-making is not the scientific evidence regarding disease pathogenesis or treatment mechanisms but rather the best empirical predictors of patient risk and factors that reduce risk." How can one know whether a treatment is biologically effective, and not a placebo, unless it has been the object of a randomized trial, double-blind and placebo-controlled, involving a large and heterogeneous sample? Besides, the concept of "empirical risk predictor" is fuzzy; it is neither mathematical nor statistical. Lastly, the results of laboratory tests are usually of a higher quality than those of massive clinical trials, because the former are conducted by trained scientists, whereas the typical massive clinical trial rests on forms filled by medical practitioners without research experience.

In a much-cited article, the philosopher John Worrall (2002) has worked out the criticism of the Bayesian Dennis Lindley, of the assumption that the RCTs discards *all* the misleading factors, both known and unknown — the *confounding factors*. This objection is correct, but it only confirms two theses, neither of which invalidates the RCTs. Let us see.

One of the thesis is that *there is no fool-proof test*, but that every test design can be improved to include previously overlooked variables. The other thesis is that, however rigorous a clinical test may be, it is *insufficient* to validate a therapy; we should also disclose the most plausible mechanism(s) of action, as Flexner (1910) had proposed in his admirable report. So, neither of the two above objections justifies giving up the gold standard, and replacing experiment with observation, clinical experience, or intuition.

Other Bayesians (or subjectivists, or personalists) have raised further objections to the RCT. They claim that, once their approach is adopted, probabilities can be estimated with or without randomization and for any number of patients, even a single one, since personal probabilities are measures of belief intensities. The pecuniary advantage of such procedure for industry is immense, as great as replacing pharmacologists with sooth-sayers. Let us hope serious pharmaceutical businessmen will keep boasting about their labs and their reliance on objective science rather than on divination. (More on subjective probabilities in Bunge 2012a.)

The preceding does not prove that the RCTs are error-free. It is well known that statistical errors of two kinds can occur: Type I (*false positives*) and Type II (*false negatives*). Examples of false positives: the therapies and drugs that had to be discontinued, after having passed RCTs, because eventually clinical practice showed that they were ineffective or even harmful. Examples of false negatives: the therapies that were prematurely rejected because they had failed preclinical trials, but were finally adopted when shown to have a beneficial mechanism of action.

What is to be done when an error of either type is discovered? Should medics go back to the casuistry that Claude Bernard consigned to the dust-bin of history? Of course not: what must be done is to reanalyze, redesign, and redo the test. Regrettably, in recent times, it has become increasingly difficult to publish replications of previous studies, even when they are shown to have yielded false findings, as often happens in psychology and psychiatry (Yong 2012). This is a serious flaw in the current peer review practice.

Scientific errors are corrected with more research, not less. And meth-odological errors, such as believing that observational studies are superior to their experimental counterparts, are corrected with more pro-science philosophy, not with phobosophies, that is, philosophies that obstruct the advancement of knowledge.

The EBM (evidence-based medicine) school swears by the *meta-analyses* of RCTs, which use statistical techniques for collating large numbers of primary RCTs, to estimate the "effective size" of a given treatment. Such analyses of primary analyses have been subjected to many criticisms, some valid but others invalid. In my opinion, the only valid objection to such second-degree analyses is that they are confined to the reports on the alleged *results* of the primary studies: these are tacitly assumed to be correct.

Now, this assumption has been seriously questioned since John Ioannidis (2005), a Stanford professor of medicine, released his bombshell: *most published research findings are false* because they had methodological flaws of some kind or other. He thus reminded us that adding zeroes only results in zero. In other words, a meta-analysis is valuable only if it involves the prior weeding out of methodologically dubious primary studies. But nearly everybody, including the EBM champions, still take meta-analyses at their face value. More on this below.

Let us conclude with three philosophical remarks on related matters. The first concerns the belief that the goal of an RCT is to evaluate the *probability* of hypotheses of the form "Therapy *T* is effective." Sometimes, it is added that, as Rudolf Carnap (1950) and others have claimed, there are two possible and equally valid interpretations of mathematical probability: the objective (as relative frequency) and the subjective (as credence or strength of belief) ones. In other words, Bayesianism and frequentism are put on a par.

However, both views are wrong for the following reasons. First, the *interpretation* of a symbol is not the same as the *evaluation* of a function. Indeed, one may use frequencies to *evaluate* probabilities, without accepting the *interpretation* (or conception) of probability as long-run frequency, just as clocks are used to measure times without necessarily accepting the operationist definition of time as "what clocks measure" (see Bunge 2012b). Hence, it is mistaken to call 'frequentist' the RCT.

Second, the frequentism/Bayesianism dilemma does not occur in the mature sciences, where a probability value quantifies the *objective possibility* or likelihood of an individual fact (state or event) *picked at random*. For example, for facts of any kind, the probability of the simultaneous occurrence of two mutually independent random facts is smaller than the probability of either of them. Note that the words 'frequency' and 'belief' are absent from the previous sentence. The reasons are that (a) frequencies are properties of collections of facts, not of individual facts, whether random or not; and (b) beliefs are brain states, hence objects of study of psychology (recall Chapter 4). Hence, there can be no *Bayesian* RCTs; these are all statistical (in particular actuarial). What does happen is that the confusion between 'probabilistic,' 'statistical,' and 'Bayesian' is rampant in the recent medical literature. And yet, if questioned, any self-styled Bayesian medic is likely to admit that medicine is about sick people rather than about the mental processes undergone by their physicians.

Our second philosophical remark is that the RCTs involve the notion of *objective chance*, in particular of random sampling. And this notion is as alien to classical (or causal) determinism as to subjectivism, in particular Bayesianism. Randomization concerns the means, not the objective of the RCT; its goal is to find out whether, and to what extent, a hypothesis is *true*, and the concept of (objective) truth is independent of that of probability. For example, it is true that an appendectomy prevents appendicitis because it excises the organ that can get infected. But it makes no sense to talk about the *probability* that the said operation has the desired effect, because this is not a random event.

Truth and its dual, falsehood, are properties of propositions or statements, whereas in the sciences and technologies, probabilities are properties of facts. A given fact may be real or imaginary, and more or less probable, but it can be neither true nor false. On the other hand, a proposition of the form "The probability of fact f is p" may be true or false to some degree. The concept of real probability is ontological (it refers to the world), whereas that of truth is epistemological or semantical (referring to our knowledge of the world or our discourse about it).

Our third and last philosophical remark is this: no experimental trial, however rigorous, can prove that a strong statistical correlation constitutes a causal link. To prove the existence of such a link, one must perform laboratory experiments showing that there has been an *energy gradient* between two things, or between two parts of a thing. In other words, we may claim that there is causation if, and only if, a *mechanism of action*, such as the bactericidal effect of an antibiotic, has been at work.

In sum, we uphold the ruling opinion that the RCT is the *gold standard* of biomedical research; it is the most objective and impartial, hence also the most reliable and responsible, method for assessing the effectiveness of medical interventions on members of heterogeneous populations.

Those who reject the RCT should also dispense with the valuable services it has performed. But those who hold that passing an RCT is both necessary and sufficient to validate a therapy are stuck in empiricism, or the cult of empirical data. This applies in particular to the clinical studies seeking only to establish statistical correlations. One such recent and much-publicized study is Vickers' (2012) meta-analysis of 29 clinical trials on the supposed benefit of acupuncture to chronic pain patients. The 17,922 subjects of the study were chosen only because they shared symptoms, from back pain to migraine, which of course may have multiple causes, from tendonitis to arthritis to stress. More precisely, the population under study was composed of people suffering from four different diseases: back and neck pain, osteoarthritis, chronic headache, and shoulder pain. (Pain, like fever, is not a disease but a symptom of many different diseases, which is why "painkillers" may alleviate but not cure.) Also, different procedures were employed, from needle to laser. So, the improvements reported in the primary literature analyzed by Vickers and coworkers point to the miracle rather than the panacea. Let us look at it a bit closer.

The Vickers *et al.* meta-analysis concerns *different diseases treated with closely related yet different therapies* — hardly the one disease-one therapy case typical of the rigorous trial aiming at checking the therapeutic effectiveness of a single therapy for a single ailment. Moreover, the trials under consideration were one-eyed rather than double-blind, for the subjects could feel whether the needles were applied by hand or electrically. In short, the Vickers study did not even meet the silver standard; it only served to prop up an ancient superstition. Ignoring mechanisms, the way biostatisticians and epidemiologists tend to do, amounts to groping in the dark.

That RCTs are necessary but insufficient to attain medical truths, if only because they may be wrongly executed, should be obvious, particularly after the highly respected and widely read *PLoS* medical journal published John Ioannidis' (2005) study, "Why most published research findings [in medicine] are false." Ioannidis listed the key factors in such a poor yield: "a research finding is less likely to be true when the studies conducted in a field are smaller; when effect sizes are smaller; when there is a greater number and lesser preselection of tested relationships; where there is greater flexibility in designs, definitions, outcomes, and analytical modes; when there is greater financial and other interest and prejudice; and when more teams are involved in a scientific field in chase of statistical significance."

Presumably, such factors lose significant weight when the RCTs are conducted primarily to check hypotheses concerning *mechanisms* that sound plausible in light of sound basic science. For instance, it is implausible that listening to music causes influenza, although hundreds of studies might well show a positive correlation between listening to music in poorly aired concert halls, with or without music, and catching the flu. The said correlation, if it were to exist, would be spurious because there is no conceivable mechanism whereby music *per se* can transmit viruses. In short, to prove that *A* causes *B*, one must exhibit the mechanism linking *A* to *B*.

Coda

In modern science and technology, it is not enough to frame explanatory hypotheses; it is also required that these be shown to be true, at least to a first approximation. And to accomplish this, it is necessary to subject hypotheses to tests of two kinds: conceptual and experimental. What I call a *conceptual test* of a hypothesis consists in showing that, far from being arbitrary, it is consistent with the bulk of the relevant antecedent knowledge. For example, no biomedical researcher would expect hints from superior beings, or check his prognoses with a soothsayer.

As for the *experimental control* of hypotheses concerning members of homogeneous populations, such as groups of molecules of the same species, or one of clones (or individuals with roughly the same genome), an experiment consists in dividing the given group into two, wiggling the variable(s) of interest in one of the groups, and comparing the resulting difference, if any. But if the original population is *heterogeneous* (with a great "variety" or diversity), as is the case in medicine, the assignment of individuals to each group must be made at random to avoid biases, as argued above.

I submit that *the gold standard is necessary but insufficient*, for it *overlooks mechanisms*. When the mechanisms of action are not well known, it is impossible to ascertain whether the presence or absence of a certain factor is a cause of bad health or a marker of it. For example, we still do not know for sure whether vitamin D prevents diseases, let alone what is the adequate dose of it. This is because it is not yet well known how it acts; the alleged benefits of vitamin D have been touted on the sole basis of observational studies, and even these have been inconclusive. This is why five massive RCTs on the effectiveness of vitamin D, involving tens of thousands of individuals, are to be conducted at different places between 2017 and 2020 (Kupferschmidt 2012).

Regrettably, none of these studies includes a close look at the manner in which vitamin D binds with its receptor. Is this omission due to a philosophical bias toward the empiricist epistemology? We won't know for sure unless a massive RCT on the philosophical attitudes of biomedical researchers is conducted. But who would dare write a grant proposal to this effect?

I propose calling *platinum standard* the dual control, conceptual and experimental, involving randomization, double-blind, and placebo, as well as the explicit statement of the mechanism of action conjectured to be at work. The platinum standard crowns the so-called trials hierarchy.

In conclusion, we may distinguish four levels of rigor in biomedical research:

Clay standard: traditional casuistry;
Silver standard: non-RCT;
Gold standard: RCT; and
Platinum standard: RCT + mechanism(s) of action.

However, even platinum can oxidize; flaws can always occur, and a good trial will culminate in a research project that, if not trivial, will raise new questions that deserve being investigated. This is one of the differences between scientific research, an open process, and pseudoscience, an ossified belief system. Whereas the "true believer" in a CAM is satisfied with a friend's testimonial ("It worked for me and for Aunt Mary"), the person who prefers the scientific approach to medical problems will appreciate, though not idolize, the tentative results of trials fitting the platinum standard.

In short, if you seek health, refuse therapies that have not undergone rigorous tests. The time has come to look at some of the philosophical issues raised by therapies.

CHAPTER 7

THERAPY

7.1 Treatment

The magical and religious worldviews discourage the search for medical treatment because they hold that sickness is punishment for sin or offense, whence only sacrifice or charm may cure it. This is how the ancient Peruvians conceived of disease — it was divine punishment. Hence, the sick person, and likewise the father of a sick child, were taken to be bad persons deserving contempt and neglect. This is why in ancient Peru, sick people were left to fend for themselves; they had to seek the help of magician-healers, who, unlike the teachers or *amautas*, held a low social rank (Valdizán 2005).

Most people in modern societies, by contrast, regard diseases as natural facts (recall Chapters 2 and 3). This is why medical treatments are sought and practiced in these societies, and also why medics are held in high esteem, though less so than wealth owners or managers. So much so, that until the nuclear scare in 1945, in ordinary language 'physician' was the synonym of 'scientist.' Also, since then, some people regard doctors as tools of Big Pharma. This distorted view of the medical profession fails to explain why so many talented people devote their lives to learning, applying, or improving ever more sophisticated therapies.

Nowadays, most people take it for granted that there is, actually or potentially, a therapy for every disease. This is certainly a more-or-less explicit principle of scientific medicine. It is not an axiom but a programmatic or heuristic hypothesis, and an extremely fertile one. Yet, it is not obvious, as proved by the variety of opinions on the matter recorded by historians: see Table 7.1.

Table 7.1. Therapy/disease pairs.

School	Therapeutic principle
Nihilism	There are no cures: sit back and watch.
Monism	A single therapy (panacea) fits all diseases.
Eclecticism	Use various therapies for every disease.
Isomorphism	One disease-one therapy, and conversely.

Therapeutic nihilism is the medical partner of radical skepticism, or the thesis that truth is either unattainable or unimportant. It is also part of naturism, and a popular reaction to the purge-and-bleed medical school ridiculed by Molière in the mid-seventeenth century. Homeopathy and acupuncture are the most popular panaceas. Many patients combine scientific medicine with CAMs (complementary and alternative medicines). Therapeutic isomorphism is the ideal of scientific medicine, but most medics practice therapeutic eclecticism when the available therapies are incomplete or have adverse or side effects. For example, antihypertensive drugs are usually combined with diuretics.

A *therapy*, or disease-treatment strategy, is a procedure for treating a disease in a professional and efficient manner. Therapy is to treatment what map is to territory. Note the key word, *efficiency*, or high output/input ratio, to be distinguished from *effectiveness*. Irradiation and chemotherapy are highly effective in destroying malignant cells, but they are inefficient because they involve the direct or indirect destruction of much healthy tissue. Efficiency, by contrast, combines effectiveness with safety and economy. And it is of course the ultimate goal of technology. Hence, those who design therapies are craftsmen in prescientific medicine, and technologists in scientific medicine.

Scientific therapies are not any old rules; unlike their predecessors, scientific therapies are based on (factual) truth, or adequacy of idea to fact, not just on custom, intuition, or experience. In particular, the search for therapies is conducted in light of findings in the biomedical sciences. Indeed, scientific medicine adopts the following bridge between efficiency and truth: *If therapy T truly weakens the causes of disease D while strengthening those of the recovery from D, as shown by controlled clinical trials of T, then T is effective and safe to treat D.* Evidently, the postmoderns, like Michel Foucault and his ilk, have no use for this criterion, because they dismiss the very concept of objective truth.

In contemporary medicine, the treatment of a sick person follows a *protocol* or plan that specifies both the therapy and the manner in which it is to be applied to that particular individual. A responsible physician will not embrace the libertarian ideology that rejects all planning; he knows that rational action is planned rather than spontaneous or improvised. But, far from being paternalistic as in the past, the contemporary doctor will ask for the informed consent of the patient, and he will be willing to discuss the protocol and even the therapy if the patient's condition does not improve as forecast. That is, nowadays, medical planning is both participative and flexible.

The practice of involving the patient in the choice of treatment is often called *patient-based medicine*, and it has been announced as a revolution in medicine (Dubertret 2006). Actually, that is no novelty in treating chronic patients, particularly those suffering from visible ailments, such as facial deformities, that hamper social intercourse to the point of requiring elective surgery. Authentic revolutions take more than changes in emphasis.

All the medical schools, at all times, have taken for granted that diseases have causes, and can be treated in some way or other. We write 'treated,' not 'cured,' because there are still incurable ailments. Some of them, such as advanced cirrhosis, multiple sclerosis, and large brain damage, are incurable because they involve irreversible losses. Presumably, other diseases are only refractory today because of insufficient medical knowledge — a condition curable by more research. Among them, the common cold, diabetes, and asthma stand out. Although their etiologies are fairly well known, no effective means to derail their courses has yet been invented.

The two hypotheses that have just been stated — on etiology and on treatment — are *causal*. And both are empirically testable, provided they involve neither supernatural powers nor paranormal abilities. In fact, biomedical research seeks to find out *natural* (or *social*) causes, as well as to devise *material* (neither supernatural nor spiritual) treatments. By contrast, invoking the supernatural, paranormal, or immaterial is the philosophical characteristic of primitive medicine (recall Chapter 1).

As soon as it is assumed that diseases and treatments are causal processes, two philosophical problems emerge: how to elucidate the notion of causation, and how to put a causal hypothesis to the test. The former problem is ontological (about things), whereas the second is methodological (about the search for truth).

The standard solution to the ontological problem in question is to conceive of the causal nexus as the relation between events whereby the cause produces the effect. More precisely, if C and E describe two events or changes, and C is prior to E, or simultaneous with E, C will be said to *cause E* if and only if C is both necessary and sufficient for E to happen ($C \Leftrightarrow E$). (See Table 7.2.)

The simplest criterion for ascertaining whether a fact of type C causes a fact of type E is to prevent the occurrence of C and check whether, in fact, E fails to happen. That is, one applies the ancient principle *Causa cessante, tollitur effectus*. In this case, if E always follows C, the causal hypothesis is

Table 7.2. Examples of causal relations.

Sufficient cause	Effect
Innate photopigments deficiency	Daltonianism
Intake of high arsenic dose	Death
Beheading	Cessation of mental processes

Necessary cause	Effect
Unprotected coition	Pregnancy
Koch bacillus	Tuberculosis
Speed ingestion	Amphetaminic psychosis

Necessary and sufficient cause	
0.2% or more alcohol in the blood	Drunkenness
Hunger in childhood	Retarded development
Prolonged dehydration	Death

Change that is neither necessary nor sufficient to get sick or cured	
Body cooling	Common cold
Cupping	Circulation stimulation
Religious conversion	Cure of any disease

confirmed; and if C happens but E does not, the hypothesis is confuted. This, confirming or refuting a causal hypothesis, is what is gained when one subjects it to a controlled experiment. As we saw in the previous chapter, an experiment is a process whereby the experimental group (on which C acts) is compared with the control group (where C does not act).

With very few exceptions, such as the experiments performed by Paracelsus, Lynd, and Jenner, traditional physicians did not perform controlled experiments, but just compared the state of health of their patients before and after treatment. That is, they indulged the classical fallacy *post hoc, ergo propter hoc* ("after this, therefore because of this"). This is a fallacy because (a) the fact taken to be the cause of a disease may be necessary or sufficient but not both; and (b) the improvement may have been spontaneous or a placebo effect — one that, though real, may not have been effected by the treatment but by the patient's belief in its effectiveness. For example, cooling won't contribute to catching the common cold without the help of the rhinovirus. Much suffering over centuries would have been avoided if barbarous treatments, like bloodletting, had been subject to experimental control centuries sooner; it would have been found that bloodletting is indicated only for acute heart failure, to reduce the venous blood overload.

The healer, herbalist, and traditional Oriental medic promised to *cure any ailment*. But they could not keep their promises, because their treatments were not backed by any experiments. Still, they had some success in prophylaxis, in nursing wounds and infections, obstetrics, plastic surgery, setting bones, and implanting dental prostheses. They could not accomplish more for lack of knowledge and excess of superstition. Their patients improved sometimes thanks to their interventions, and at others despite them, and always spontaneously — courtesy of their immune systems — or through placebo effects. But they were often the victims of superstitions, such as the belief, held in Spain until about 1600, that a wound healed as it secreted pus, which is why the medic would enlarge it.

The healer and the traditional doctor commanded enormous prestige, not only because of the enormous and arcane knowledge attributed to him, but also because of the moral support he lent his patients. He earned their gratitude, respect, obedience, and even affection, because of his concern for them. When the shaman doubled as chief, his prestige as healer gave him also political clout. That is, knowledge, whether genuine or imaginary, gave power.

The social prestige of those who promised the recovery of health was comparable to that of the wealth owner or the powerful leader. He often sat at the prince's table. Nowadays, the physician is a well-respected crafts-man, and occasionally better paid than a plumber, though never as well as a banker. And his social status differs from one country to the next. Whether self-employed or in the pay of a health care organization, the typical physician is overworked, so that he will have hardly any time left to update his knowledge. He depends largely on pharmaceutical repre-sentatives to keep up with medical advances.

The contemporary physician promises far less than the healer but accomplishes far more. In fact, he does not promise to heal, much less to "save lives," that is, postpone deaths, but only to assist, alleviate, and advise. In discharging this task, sometimes he succeeds in controlling the course of disease, sometimes healing, and always alleviating. To do all that, he draws from the body of medical knowledge that has been growing spectacularly since about 1850, particularly since the birth of experimental medicine, bacteriology, pharmacology, and surgery, as well as the powerful pharmaceutical industry born around 1900.

There is a tendency to ignore everything published before the personal computer. Thus, as we saw in Chapter 2, it is becoming fashionable to equate the birth of scientific medicine with the start of the so-called evidence-based medicine (or practice), or EBM, around 1990 (e.g., Sackett *et al.* 1996; Dawes *et al.* 2005). But medicine proper, unlike shamanism and traditional Oriental medicine, has always relied on evidence, and particularly so since the 1500s (recall Chapter 2). What is true is that medicine has become far more effective since the invention of antibiotics and the randomized controlled trial (RCT).

Still, a therapy that has approved all the phases of a rigorous RCT will fail in some cases, because in every population of organisms there are some exceptional individuals. (In clinical trials, such outliers are likely to be discarded as experimental errors.) For example, it may happen that an individual has a mutation in a tumor-suppressing gene, so that the anti-carcinogens he is getting do not work. When such genetic failures are suspected, genetic sequencing might be indicated, so that the therapy can be "personalized," that is, tailored to the individual's genome. However, there is no evidence yet that such knowledge will result in health gains (Nebert & Zhang 2012).

While praising the accomplishments of contemporary therapy, we should not forget its spectacular failures (see Groopman 2008). Here is a glimpse of this gallery of horrors: lobotomy, which cut out free will; hysterectomy, which Charcot, the young Freud's hero, practiced to cure "hysteria"; defenestration, recommended to recover hearing, but which unnecessarily destroyed large parts of the internal ear; mastectomy and the removal and fusion of lumbar vertebrae, which turned out to be unnecessary most times; pneumothorax (lung collapse), often used to treat lung tuberculosis with uncertain results other than creating surgical fame; tonsillectomy, which removed a useful gland, in most cases unnecessarily; electroshock, that was used liberally to relieve depression even though nobody knew how it worked; and hormone replacement to "cure" menopause, but which was found to be harmful on balance. No doubt, all of these highly invasive therapies were imaginative and had some basis. But they had not been subjected to RCTs, and violated the precautionary principle.

The *precautionary principle* is the rule according to which one should always prefer the intervention (or the inaction) bringing more benefit than harm. That is, before adopting a course of action (or inaction), we should try to estimate its *net value* — the difference between its benefits and risks. For example, chemotherapy is generally successful at the beginning of a cancer growth, but it is useless and therefore cruel in the advanced stages. Much the same holds for all other invasive tests, such as endoscopies, biopsies, and X-rays — there can be too much of them (Welch *et al.* 2011).

Although the words *benefit* and *harm* (or *risk*) sound self-explanatory, it is not clear how to measure, or even identify, the corresponding variables. Shorter: we do not know how to objectively and exactly evaluate the net benefit or harm of a therapy. It is often said that it equals the amount of enjoyable life it causes us to gain or lose. This would be reasonable if we had the relevant statistical data. But all these tell us is, at best, how much time a given therapy adds or subtracts *on average* in populations of a given type. And this lapse of time is a *collective* trait, not an individual one. Hence knowledge of it, though valuable, does not help much in making individual prognoses.

The only field where it is known how to measure risks are those of the games of chance, where the risk of a bet or investment equals the amount of it times the probability of losing. But what are such amounts and probabilities in the case of health and disease? These are states, not magnitudes, and they have to do with causation, not chance. Assigning them probabilities amounts to mistaking clinics for casinos.

Besides, the benefits of a therapy are often immediate but, as a treatment is prolonged, adverse effects may start to appear, and by then the treatment has been applied to a large number of patients. Let's face it: the search for effective and safe treatments, as well as for reasonably exact prognoses, is still on the agenda of biomedical research, and it is likely to remain there.

In conclusion, therapies and the correlative clinical decisions come in several degrees of reliability:

1) *Negative*: It assumes impossible mechanisms (e.g., magical) or has failed rigorous trials. *Discard.*
2) *Null*: lacking in both biological plausibility and experimental support. *Suspend both judgment and use.*
3) *Very weak*: biologically plausible but not yet subjected to trial. *Refrain from applying but subject to stringent tests.*
4) *Weak*: passed rigorous tests but has no known mechanism of action. *Adopt pro tempore but keep testing.*
5) *Strong*: known mechanism of action and validated by RCTs. *Adopt but keep looking for possible adverse effects.*

Here are a few examples:

1) In 1889, the physiologist Oskar Minkowski discovered that the ablation of the pancreas causes diabetes. Thereafter, research on diabetes concentrated on that organ, and culminated with the discovery and therapeutic use of insulin by Frederick Banting and Charles Best in 1921.
2) Defective heart valves can be replaced with artificial ones, because their role is purely hydraulic: to interrupt and restore the flow of blood.

3) The pill that dilates the airways can also be used to prevent esophageal spasms because it works as a muscle relaxant.

4) Cryotherapy is based on the finding that exposure to intense cold for a short time causes well-being — it is "invigorating" as Canadians say — although actually it is debilitating. That is because exposure to cold activates circulation, metabolism, and the synthesis of endorphins (brain-made analgesics).

5) Bactericides cure by killing pathogens or blocking either their metabolism or their multiplication.

The preceding cases instantiate the rule *Prefer the therapy with a known mechanism of action and that best passes RCTs*. In Chapter 6, we called this convention the *platinum standard* for regarding it superior to the gold standard, or approval of an RCT. But of course, effective and safe therapies should be used even if their mechanisms of action are still unknown.

The case of aspirin is exemplary: it was used successfully as an analgesic, anti-inflammatory, and blood-thinner over seven decades without knowledge of its mechanism of action. In fact, it was only in 1971 that the pharmacologist John Vane revealed this in his paper in *Nature*, titled "Inhibition of prostaglandin synthesis as a mechanism of action for aspirin-like drugs." But, as found only recently, a high price was paid by the blind use of aspirin; in fact, aspirin overdose has been blamed for the death of up to 100 million people during the Spanish influenza pandemic following the First World War (recall Section 5.2).

Research on mechanisms of action has both a practical and a philosophical justification. Practical because, to act efficiently on a system, we must control not only its input, but also its intervening mechanism, since any given cause will have different effects when acting on different mechanisms: see Figure 7.1. And the philosophical justification for research on

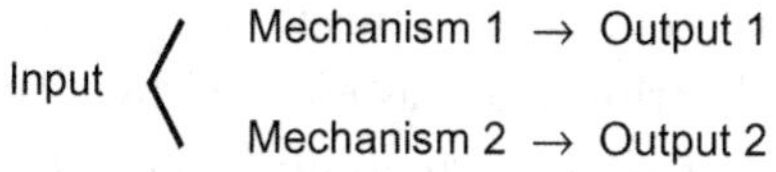

$$\text{Input} \left\{ \begin{array}{l} \text{Mechanism 1} \rightarrow \text{Output 1} \\ \text{Mechanism 2} \rightarrow \text{Output 2} \end{array} \right.$$

Fig. 7.1. One and the same input may trigger different outputs when acting on two different systems, or on two different mechanisms in the same system.

mechanisms is that explaining a fact consists in revealing the manner in which it is produced (Bunge 2006).

Explanations in terms of mechanisms do not abound in medicine, and most of them were found only after the Second World War. Thus, writing of his internship in 1937, Lewis Thomas (1983: 42) reminisces that "lobar pneumonia is the only disease I can remember that had an intellectually satisfying explanation for what went on." The mechanism was the lung's invasion by pneumococci, which provoked an immune reaction that the doctor could boost by injecting an antibody (a rabbit's serum) whose molecular configuration matched precisely that of the bacterium. Thus, the treatment matched the dynamics or mechanism of the disease.

Newton taught us that *kinematics*, the description of motion, never suffices; we should also try to learn why things move the way they do — that is, *dynamics*. For example, the cardiologist needs to know not only that blood circulates, but also what makes it move and what may alter its motion, so that he may know what to do in the case of circulation trouble. (After all, the main journal of the American Heart Association is called *Circulation*.) And the hematologist must also know something about the generation and composition of blood — for example, that leukemia is due to a low production rate of red blood cells from stem cells in the bone marrow, so that only radical therapies, such a chemotherapy and bone marrow transplant, may cure it.

This principle, that we should know not only *what* happens but also *why* it happens or fails to happen, sounds obvious to us, but it was emphatically denied by the positivist philosophers and the scientists they influenced. In particular, the eminent physicists Ernst Mach (aerodynamics) and Gustav Kirchhoff (spectroscopy) taught that scientists should describe, not explain. Descriptivism was so influential between 1850 and 1950 that, when some logical positivists finally accepted explanation, they reduced it to the logical operation of subsuming the particular under the general — the so-called nomological-deductive model — instead of centering on mechanisms. (The core of this idea was that a fact was explained if the proposition F describing it was entailed by a law statement L conjoined with the circumstances C attending F, such as the initial conditions: $L \ \& \ C \vdash F$. This Pickwickian analysis was alien to the notions of explanation prevailing since Aristotle.)

We close this section by listing some of the philosophical ideas that any scientific physician takes for granted when treating a patient:

1) The patient exists really in the doctor's external world.
2) Diseases are real and natural processes, not social conventions.
3) All diseases can in principle be known, even though some of them are not well known, or even suspected, due to the imperfections of today's medicine.
4) All diseases, except for the purely imaginary ones, are manifested as objective signs, and sometimes also as symptoms that only the sick person may feel. While different diseases may have the same symptoms, there is one bundle of signs for every disease.
5) Every piece of effective therapeutic knowledge is an objective truth, though possibly only a partial or approximate one.
6) All diseases are treatable, i.e., susceptible of being altered by medical interventions, but only some of them are curable with currently available means.
7) Every treatment consists in manipulating real properties, and this occurs even in the case of logotherapies, such as the shamanic, religious, and psychotherapeutic ones. This is so because the perceived word, image, and gesture impact on the brain. In turn, some of the patient's mental processes affect his health because they modify his behavior or his immune system. This is why optimists are likely to recover faster than pessimists.
8) All therapies are artificial (man-made); none are natural, even if they employ only natural products, since every treatment, even if purely symptomatic, is made and interferes with the natural course of the disease. However, there are also some iatrogenic diseases, that is, disorders caused involuntarily by wrong medical interventions or by unsanitary conditions in hospitals or frontline medical outfits.
9) While some therapies are superficial or "sweet," others are radical or invasive; and whereas most of the former are purely symptomatic, the latter affect the underlying mechanisms, most of which are imperceptible for being molecular (like cancer) or cellular (like viral infections). For example, the newest drugs to treat hepatitis C act effectively and quickly because they attack the virus directly.

10) The superficial therapies are typical of the prescientific medicines, whereas the radical ones, like root canal, thoracic surgery, and biological psychiatry, have been designed with the help of biology and have aimed at the root of the trouble. For example, some hematological diseases may require chemotherapy or sophisticated surgery to quicken the generation of hematopoietic (blood-generating) stem cells. In short, in medicine, as elsewhere, we must distinguish peel from pulp. This distinction, inherent in scientific realism, is denied by the anti-realist philosophies, such as subjectivism, phenomenalism, fictionism, and conventionalism.

7.2 Placebo, Panacea, Resistance

The placebo effects, which used to be themes of anecdotes and stories, are now topical research problems in psychology, neuroscience, and medicine (Benedetti 2009). Two distinct components of a placebo effect should be distinguished: object and response. A *placebo object* is a thing or procedure that alleviates an ailment without acting directly on the organism; its effect is called the *placebo response*. In short, a placebo effect can be analyzed as the ordered pair <*object, response*>. Maybe the shaman's ritual had a more beneficial effect than the product he sold. A more subtle placebo is the affectionate and encouraging smile of the traditional family doctor.

The placebo response is real, though it is not due to the placebo object but to the patient's belief in its effectiveness, that is, his expectation (Kirsch 1985). If the expectation is negative, one talks about a *nocebo*. For these reasons, it has been called "the belief effect." This name is justified because the effect disappears when the subject realizes that she has been lied to. It also disappears when the patient is given naloxone, a drug used to treat substance abuse.

At first sight, the placebo effect supports the dualist belief in the power of the immaterial mind over the material body. Actually, it does just the opposite. Indeed, recent studies with fMRI (functional magnetic resonance imaging) have shown that a placebo object activates the same brain regions that are stimulated with opiates, among them the endorphins synthesized by the brain itself. That is, the placebo response is a brain process.

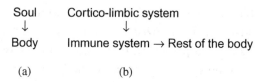

Fig. 7.2. Two contrasting views of high/low and of psychosomatic medicine: (a) psychoneural dualism (mind over matter); and (b) psychoneural monism (thinking matter here over unthinking matter there).

Still, the placebo response may be regarded as an instance of a *top-down* process occurring at the border between the cognitive and the emotive. However, the "higher" is not the immaterial soul but the cerebral cortex in close contact with its social environment; and the "lower" is composed of subcortical organs, among them the nucleus accumbens, or pleasure center, and the amygdala, or fear center (Lane *et al.* 2009). (See Figure 7.2.)

The belief associated with the placebo effect does not arise spontaneously; it only occurs in a brain manipulated by the persons who offer the placebo object. And the response is stronger the greater the prestige or authority of the professional, whether medic or priest. Besides, the more expensive the placebo objects are, the more effective they turn out to be — as was to be expected in a consumer society.

Let us emphasize that the placebo *response* occurs in the brain, so that the object–response pair is a *biosocial* fact. This alone recommends it for a greater attention on the part of neuroscientists and psychologists, particularly those with a sociological inclination. As suggested above, it is likely that the placebo response occurs in the cortico-limbic, or cognition–emotion frontier. But, since this answer is too imprecise, the problem is still under research.

The above is highly relevant to the RCT, studied in the previous chapter. Indeed, such a trial does not suffice to ascertain that a certain therapy is a placebo object, because *all* therapies, whether well grounded or phony, have a placebo effect. To make sure that a drug has *only* such an effect, that is, that it has no pharmacodynamic (chemical or biological) effect, it must be subjected to chemical or biological assays in a test tube or a Petri dish. Again, appearances are not enough; we must get down to the nitty-gritty of the biological mechanisms presumably at play.

Hypnosis, which can be induced by a person vested with authority of some kind, is similar. The hypnotized subject looks relaxed, expectant, and willing to cooperate — in particular, to assume the roles assigned him by the hypnotist. (Something similar happens to the Japanese macaque in relation to the experimenter, whom he obeys as if he were the alpha male.) But there is no such thing as a hypnotic "trance" or zombie state, despite the prosperity of the zombie industry in the current philosophy of mind. Nor is it true that the hypnotized subject can be forced to do something against his own will — for example, to kill on behalf of the hypnotizer.

On the other hand, it is true that "mass hysteria," or large-scale suggestion, can be provoked by a charismatic leader. In fact, the social psychologists Solomon Asch, Albert Bandura, Leo Festinger, Stanley Milgram, and Muzafer Sherif showed several decades ago that an individual surrounded by a band of fanatics or of accomplices of the experimenter is more easily suggestible than an isolated individual, particularly an insecure one.

It is well known that there are different degrees of suggestibility, hence of gullibility; there are "good" subjects and others who resist suggestion. (I am skeptical, you are naïve, and he is a fanatic.) It has been suggested that susceptibility to suggestion, as to anything else, is partially hereditary, and that it is reinforced or weakened during childhood. But, like so many questions in the nature/nurture field, this one is still unresolved. However, back to placebos.

All health workers, whether or not scientific, count on the placebo effect even if they do not use it deliberately. The first stage of a placebo effect is cognitive (belief and expectancy). But, if we admit that everything mental is cerebral, and that the brain is intimately connected with the immune and endocrine systems, it should not be surprising that some beliefs have a therapeutic effect, and others a nocebo one. This is why there are placebos for pain and depression, as well as for insomnia and somnolence, but not for processes that occur without the intervention of the brain, such as cellular division and apoptosis, infection, and arthritis.

There are two common objections to treating mental disorders with pills. One is that those disorders cannot be just the result of imbalances among neurotransmitters, because connections too must matter. Of course they do; without them there would be no neural systems, but it so happens that the bridges among neurons are neurotransmitters. Another popular objection is that the use of pills discourages "talking therapies," which is wrong because humans are very sensitive to speech. This objection is redundant because most psychiatrists combine chemical therapy with cognitive therapy, or they attempt to correct bad habits as well as to instill hope. Talk can help unless it is nonsensical.

How do placebos work? Several mechanisms are known, and presumably more will soon be discovered. One of them is conditioning. For example, if a subject is given an efficient remedy in a red capsule, he may end up by associating his improvement with the color red (conditioned stimulus); therefore, the drug may eventually be replaced with a red capsule containing only an inert substance.

A second placebo effect, involved in the case of pain, is the spontaneous segregation of endogenous opiates (endorphins). A third is the synthesis of dopamine, the "happy hormone." A creationist might claim that all this proves that we have been designed with intelligence and compassion. By contrast, an evolutionist will argue that those who feel unwell all the time do not reproduce, so that their lineage tends to become extinct.

The placebo effect is related to *cognitive control*, another top-down process known since antiquity but investigated only in recent times. A popular example is the control that yogis and fakirs exert on their heart and metabolic rates (Dworkin & Miller 1986). The key to explaining the willed control of certain visceral processes is a nerve fiber, which had eluded previous anatomists, between the prefrontal cortex and the subcortical system of emotion (Ochsner & Gross 2005).

Another remarkable discovery was the confirmation of the popular belief in the "will to live": optimists recover faster than pessimists, from both illness and life blows. In this case, the key is the tenuous nerve connections among the cerebral cortex on the one hand, and the thymus, spleen, and lymph on the other (Locke & Hornig-Rohan 1983).

This research does not confirm psychoneural dualism, but rather the hypothesis of the interactions between the organ of the mind and the rest of the human body through nerves, blood, lymph, and hormones (Bunge & Ardila 2002). The medical moral is that scientific psychosomatic medicine is psycho-neuro-endocrino-immunology. However, back to the placebo.

The general lesson to be drawn from the preceding is that Doctor Placebo is always at the sick person's bedside, either to confound the physician or to help the patient. Acknowledging this fact has two practical consequences. The first is that clinical trials with human subjects should always control for placebos. That is, the experimental group should be split into two subgroups: the treated and the fooled by a placebo. Another consequence is that it is not enough for the practicing physician to choose the best (most efficient) therapy and protocol; he will also have to consider whether it is morally licit to use a placebo, such as a subtherapeutic dose, to start treating a refractory disease, such as deep clinical depression. The "alternative" healers do not face this moral problem because they do not measure anything.

The second subject of this section involves the cure-all therapies or panaceas. A *medical panacea* is, of course, a therapy recommended to treat, or even cure, all ailments, or at least all those of a genus, such as cancer. During the Middle Ages, it was common to prescribe drugs with 60 or more components, some of which turned out to be toxic. For instance, Theriac, a popular panacea, had about 100 ingredients.

The oldest panaceas are bloodletting and acupuncture, which have been practiced for two millennia. Bloodletting was practically abandoned when, in the mid-nineteenth century, it was discovered that it was innocuous in the best of cases, and harmful in the worst. By contrast, acupuncture is still being widely practiced on the sole strength of tradition. When subject to an RCT, it showed only a tiny placebo effect, even when toothpicks instead of needles were inserted at random (Cherkin *et al.* 2009; Sanz 2012).

Paracelsus, a contemporary of Martin Luther's and a bridge between medieval quackery and modern medicine, was an early critic of the very idea of a panacea. He proposed the modern hypothesis that all diseases are specific, so that their treatments too should be specific. This daring hypothesis was confirmed only half a millennium later, when Paul Ehrlich discovered and studied the drug receptors mounted on cell membranes. His first accomplishment was the discovery of how the tetanus antitoxin works. Ehrlich's research, and the sudden expansion of pharmacology that it triggered, should suffice to convince anyone that the *search for mechanism* has been the main engine of modern science.

The failure of any number of alleged panaceas over two millennia does not prove the impossibility of finding the perfect one. But the following considerations should persuade anyone that the search for the perfect panacea is just as futile as the pursuit of eternal youth.

First, there is no such thing as general disease; every disease has its own specific mechanism. Second, every therapy, except for rest and moderation, must be specific because it hinges on a mechanism of its own. Third, human beings, endowed as we are with a creative cerebral cortex, are susceptible to suggestion and delusion, so that almost any treatment is initially effective. This is also why books like *The End of Illness* are still in print.

Let us finally tackle the problem of the acquired tolerance or resistance to drugs: why some pathogens become increasingly impregnable to the most powerful drugs, such as antibiotics. In fact, once in a while, mutations in RNA or DNA give rise to new strains of bacteria and viruses that prove invulnerable to vaccines and drugs that used to be effective in fighting the original strain. Such mutations and their biological effects pose some philosophical as well as practical problems. Let us glance at them.

A philosophical problem with such mutations is this: since mutations are random, molecular biology, bacteriology, and virology use probability theory to study them. But the effects of mutated pathogens on cells are causal, not random; whereas some of them will be ineffective, others will provoke the immune system to produce the adequate antibodies, and still others will attack the body unopposed. In sum, randomness on one level of organization will induce causation in the next. This alternation of chance and cause happens in several fields, and it suggests that, although the two categories are interrelated, neither is reducible to the other (Bunge 1951).

The practical problems posed by the mutations of viruses and bacteria are formidable. Consider just two of them: the redesign of vaccines to meet the threats posed by mutants, and the effects of mutations on the production and consumption of food. Since mutations are unpredictable, the virologist must await their occurrence before attempting to redesign a vaccine to prevent people from "catching" the new variant of a given disease, such as the flu or AIDS. So, the virologist can never sleep on his laurels, but must always be ready to confront a somewhat different "enemy" — his is a sort of guerrilla warfare. Something similar happens to the industrial "translation" of virology, namely the mass production of new variants of a vaccine. Incidentally, all of the above confirms that evolution is molecular as well as organismic, and that vaccines are so effective that they may become obsolete — a paradox typical of scientific and technological progress.

As for the consequences of pathogen mutation on both therapy and food production, it suffices to recall that drug resistance is often an unanticipated effect of antibiotic abuse, especially in hospitals and animal farms. Every time we eat a product from those farms, we involuntarily ingest high doses of antibiotics given to the animals to protect them from infectious diseases, which render us increasingly resistant to those medicaments. This is only one of the unexpected sectoral business strategies that seek to maximize short-term private benefits regardless of the public good. A pro-people and science-informed government would exert a stricter control on the food industry because of its impact on health. And less timid political parties would point out that the free-market ideology is not only socially dissolving but also a health hazard.

It is high time to learn that there are social values, such as peace, public health, and disinterested inquiry, that the market cannot produce or even protect, as well as that, in a viable society, social justice consists in the fact that every right implies some duty, and conversely. For example, the right to public health care implies the duty to take good care of one's own health, and the right to procreate implies the duty to bring up one's children. If you agree that your health depends on mine, you'll cooperate with me at least on the field of public health (Bunge 2008).

7.3 The Probabilistic Siren Calls Again

If quantum theory held at all levels, as it has become popular to maintain, we would have to admit that getting sick and being cured are random processes and that, consequently, medicine is basically a probabilistic science, where probabilities — such as that of developing pneumonia after bronchitis — are calculated and measured with the help of that theory.

For better or for worse, quantum theory is of no help to biology and medicine, which handle mesoscopic things, like DNA molecules, and macrophysical ones, from the cell up; and, when they deal with atoms or molecules, these sciences conceive of them as classical things, with well-defined states, shapes, and trajectories. The typically quantum theoretical concepts of primary or uncaused chance, coherence (or superposition of states), and entanglement do not occur in biology or medicine. In particular, these sciences assume that a cell is either here or there, in this or that "sharp" state, healthy or sick — never half alive and half dead, like Schrödinger's imaginary cat.

To be sure, quantum theory is used in pharmacology via chemistry, but molecules are conceived of as balls joined by rods. Medicine starts only at the macromolecular level. And things at this level may be viewed as being, at each instant, in a "sharp" state, that is, one that is not the sum of elementary states; the parts of a system that splits into two, such as the daughters of a cell that has just divided, do not remain entangled; and in medicine, the concept of chance applies only to numerous collections of things or facts of a given kind. Moreover, the notions of organism, evolution, and disease are utterly alien to quantum theory.

It is true that there is often talk of the *probability* of getting sick or cured. But, as we saw in Sections 4.2 and 4.3, and will see again in the following, the "probabilities" in question are actually relative frequencies, and these are not logically related to chance or randomness. (Suffice it to think of the frequency with which we are expected to take a certain medication.) Again, epidemiologists use the concept of contagion probability, but only in the case of random encounters between sick and healthy individuals. Since physicians do not have probabilistic theories in etiology or in therapeutics, they should stick to frequencies, and pay no attention to the fictitious "probabilities" that the Bayesians invent, for they are nothing but belief strengths.

In recent years, there has been a spate of publications on the application of *decision theory* to medicine. The foci of this theory are the concepts of subjective probability and subjective benefit, that is, strength of belief and gain attributed to the application of the belief, respectively.

Decision theory goes back to Pascal's wager. Blaise Pascal asked about the value of belief in God, and reasoned roughly as follows. Since God's existence cannot be proved, we must wager that He does or does not exist. But in this game, contrary to the games of chance, we do not know the probability p of God's existence nor, consequently, the dual probability $1-p$ that He does not. However, our religion guarantees that, if we believe and act accordingly, we will earn eternal bliss. And the value of this option is infinite, whereas the atheist's is at best nil. These values are the weights of the corresponding probabilities. In other words, the weighted or *expected probabilities* are $p \times$ infinity and $(1-p) \times 0$, respectively. Conclusion: believing is infinitely more convenient than disbelieving, regardless of the value of the unknowable probability p.

Put in practical terms: let us ignore theological disputes, and rely on faith, for this is more convenient than either doubting or negating. Of course, this argument is utilitarian, and therefore blasphemous to any sincere believer. In any event, decision theory, born from religious anxiety, was expanded and articulated by the eminent mathematician and physicist Daniel Bernoulli nearly three centuries ago, and has been applied in microeconomics, political science, management science, military strategy, and recently in medicine as well.

The central dogma of decision theory is that, given a choice among several courses of action, every one of which has an outcome with a given probability and a given utility, the rational thing to do is to choose the one with the greatest expected utility. Since this is what some eminent mathematicians, from Daniel Bernoulli to John von Neumann, have advised, until very recently, no one had the temerity to set up experiments to check whether successful rational actors do in fact behave as prescribed.

The authors of these applications did not notice that neither of the two key concepts of the theory, those of subjective probability and subjective utility, has been well defined (Bunge 1996a, 1998a). Indeed, subjective probability, by contrast to mathematical probability, is a psychological variable whose values vary from one subject to the next, since it is nothing but strength of belief. The same or worse holds for subjective utility: what benefits the rich may harm the poor, and so on. Of course, these subjectivities are virtues in the eye of the decision theorist, but they are unforgivable sins in that of the scientist and the technologist, who are likely to point out that a variable whose values are assigned arbitrarily is not to be taken seriously, because it is not measurable in an objective fashion.

The decision-theory enthusiasts have also chosen to ignore the many empirical counterexamples proposed since the mid-twentieth century by the economist George Allais, the management scientist James March, the psychologist Daniel Kahneman, and the Zürich school of experimental economics, of Hans Fehr and colleagues. All of these researchers have found that real people do not behave the way decision theory postulates. In fact, they found that most of us are basically neither egoists nor altruists, but "strong reciprocators," that is, eager to win but also willing to help defend other people's rights (Gintis *et al.* 2005.)

However, since decision theory still has defenders in medicine, let us see how it works in this field. Call T_1 and T_2 two treatments, with success probabilities p_1 and p_2, and utilities u_1 and u_2, respectively. The consistent Bayesian (subjectivist) will make up the probability values, whereas the inconsistent one will equate them to the relative frequencies found in the medical literature. As for the therapeutic utilities, they are usually set equal to the years of life presumably gained by the treated individuals. Now that the alleged data are in, the decision theorist proceeds as follows:

Treatment T_1: Expected utility = $p_1 \cdot u_1$.
Treatment T_2: Expected utility = $p_2 \cdot u_2$.
Decision rule: Prefer T_1 to T_2 if, and only if, $p_1 \cdot u_1 > p_2 \cdot u_2$.

The simplest case is that of a very effective treatment with a high rate of success. To be more precise, suppose that $p = u = 9/10$. In this case, the expected utility is $= 9/10 \times 9/10 = 81/100 \approx 4/5$. This is a high value, hence a good strategy. But we hardly needed numbers to reach that conclusion, all the more since there is no reason to assume that treatments act at random.

Let us next apply the same rule to a problematic case: the dilemma between a very successful treatment with a poor benefit, and that of a rarely successful treatment with a high benefit. We shall pick arbitrary numerical values leading to the same expected utility in both cases:

$p_1 = 9/10$, $u_1 = 1/10$, $p_1 u_1 = 9/100$, *Low risk, low benefit.*
$p_2 = 1/10$, $u_2 = 9/10$, $p_2 u_2 = 9/100$, *High risk, high benefit.*

Obviously, in this case, the decision rule leaves us in the lurch, hence the physician must abstain from intervening. But if either he or his patient feels that something must be done, as gambling is preferable to inaction, the choice between the two treatments will depend on temperament — in particular, on whether the decision-maker is risk-averse or impetuous.

Since gambling is irrational when clean, and immoral when "fixed," there are at least three possibilities: (a) the given decision rule is simplistic, since it does not take into account such factors as recovery time, quality of life, and cost; (b) our knowledge of the probabilities and utilities involved is insufficient; and (c) the effectiveness of a treatment is not a matter of chance, for it depends on how it affects the mechanism of action in question.

Maybe all three reasons are valid, but the third should suffice to alter course: to expel decision theory from medicine, just as it has been expelled from all the other fields where it has been tried. The rational thing to do is to admit that the effectiveness of therapies hinges on the causal mechanisms they trigger, control, or block. Consequently, therapies should be evaluated in light of the mechanisms of action as well as of the outcomes of RCTs. This is the *platinum standard* (Chapter 6).

Incidentally, has the medical application of decision theory been subjected to RCTs, in the manner that the clinical/statistical dilemma was resolved for diagnosis and prognosis as reported in Section 4.2? If not, why is it still being taught? Just because numbers give it a veneer of scientificity, even though most of them are made up? Nobody can responsibly deny that medicine needs numbers, but these must result from theories or measurements, not from a stage magician's hat. Health, justice, and truth are too serious to be gambled with.

Coda

Except for some of their prophylactic and dietetic recommendations, the therapies proposed by the primitive and archaic medical schools have at best a placebo effect. This effect is real but small and short-lasting, because those treatments never attain the root causes, such as mutation, arterial obstruction, glandular deficiency, or infection.

This is not the case for the scientific therapies: these have effects that, although sometimes only symptomatic, are objective, that is, independent of the patient's beliefs. Still, most modern therapies are designed to treat diseases at an advanced state, so that sometimes the physician arrives only a few days before the undertaker. Yet, outcomes of this kind can be avoided by periodic checkups, since they can detect the early signs of most fatal diseases.

As a result of the sensational advances of scientific medicine during the last century, there remain few incurable diseases, like diabetes, multiple sclerosis, and Alzheimer's; and a number, in particular smallpox, poliomyelitis, typhus, cholera, yellow fever, Guinea worm disease, and rinderpest have all but disappeared almost everywhere. Moreover, nowadays, the venereal diseases can easily be avoided, and family size can be controlled and, consequently, the tragedy of millions of unwanted children can be averted.

But worldwide and consistent family planning practices require more than easy availability of contraceptives and abortion; they also require early sex education, which is still being opposed by influential religious and conservative political groups. It should become public knowledge that engendering children without being able to bring them up is just as criminal as torturing them. However, this task requires much more than vigorous campaigns of the sanitary authority; it also requires the collaboration of schools and voluntary associations.

Scientific medicine has made spectacular progress since its birth around 1800, but we should not declare victory in the "war" on disease. First, because the "wars" on cancer, alcoholism, substance abuse, violent behavior, and medical quackery are still ongoing. In particular, the "war" on cancer is still on. Specifically, an editorial in the *Lancet* for February 9, 2013, warned that "Current strategies to control cancer are demonstrably not working." Worse, the only important and robust finding of medical genetics, until recently the wunderkind of medicine, is that the *one disease-one gene* principle is just one more failure of genetic reductionism.

The second reason that it cannot be claimed that the "war" on disease has been won, is that the vast majority of the world population has no access to scientific medicine. For example, only one in 20 fertile women has access to contraceptive pills. Third, only 21 of 1,556 new drugs that reached the market between 1975 and 2004 targeted tuberculosis or tropical diseases such as parasitosis and dengue (Chirac & Torreele 2006). The reason is that the billion or so individuals susceptible to those diseases cannot afford to buy health. And, whereas in the prosperous regions there may be one physician for about every 200 inhabitants or less, in the poor regions there is only one for 50,000 — and that one is often an incompetent, underpaid, and uncaring civil servant.

Fourth, there are developed and emergent nations where the practice of medicine is a lucrative profession rather than a calling, so that health is a commodity. As a result, the life expectancy of a rich person is up to 20 years longer than that of a poor one. This fact raises a moral problem that ethics professors rarely face: that of the scarcity of social justice conceived as the balance between private concerns and public duties. But why should an ethics professor be bothered with this problem, if it was not discussed by any of the classical philosophers, let alone by Nietzsche, Heidegger, or Wittgenstein?

The fifth reason that the "war" on disease is yet to be won is that, wherever the practice of medicine is not regulated by the state the way the legal and engineering professions are, it may be severely distorted. Suffice it to mention the trade in organs for transplant, the artificial induction of multiparous births, the intensive care of irreversibly comatose patients and of severely premature babies who will not develop into normal adults, unnecessary Cesarean sections, overmedication, and excess of cosmetic surgery. In short, competent health care is available for the first time in history, but it is still economically inaccessible to most human beings, and occasionally it is distorted by pecuniary incentives.

Still, no one can deny that science-based medicine has made sensational advances since about 1800. They owe nothing to the most famous modern philosophers, from Kant and Hegel to Heidegger, Wittgenstein, or even Russell — the only pro-science of them. By contrast, medical progress owes much to the rationalist, realist, materialist, systemic, scientistic, and humanist philosophy sketched by the members of the radical wing of the French Enlightenment, notably d'Holbach, Helvétius, Diderot, and La Mettrie — all of them at odds with the political and academic establishments of their day. These bold thinkers indirectly stimulated biomedical research as the source of ever safer and more effective therapies. Since then, medicine, unlike quackery, has been practicing the maxim *Primum cognoscere, deinde medicari*: Learn before medicating.

CHAPTER 8

PREVENTION

8.1 Prognosis

The ancient Romans used one of two methods to prognosticate the course of a disease: the augur's and the experience of the Galenic medic. The augur or diviner "interpreted" the flight and entrails of a bird. He embraced the holistic principle that everything is strongly connected to everything else, as well as the hermeneutic principle that everything is a symbol of something else. Besides, his prophecy was couched in ambiguous terms, so that it was hard to tell whether it had been right or not.

By contrast, any disciple of Galen's knew of two great discoveries of the Hippocratic school. One was that every disease of a given type follows its own natural course, which no magic or religious rite could alter. The other discovery was that there are always two possible outcomes: recovery, which was spontaneous except in the cases of severe wounds or infections; and death, which could never be staved off with the means then available.

The Galenic medic's collection of clinical histories, both oral and written, suggested him to often and carefully examine the patient's overall appearance, as well as the color and smell of his urine and feces to guess the composition of his four humors. His procedure was rational and empirical, but not scientific, for scientific medicine emerged nearly two millennia later.

In the mature sciences and technologies, forecasts are calculated with the help of laws and empirical data. For example, to predict the time of flight of an airplane moving at a constant speed, one uses the formula "duration = distance/velocity." A pharmacologist can foresee what kind of drugs will affect a given receptor with known properties. Epidemiologists use equations allowing them to predict when an outbreak will turn into an epidemic, as well as how long the latter is likely to last.

By contrast, in individual medicine, very few laws are known, so that prognoses are cast with the help of different methods. The two most common are the clinical and the statistical ones. The *clinical* or intuitive method uses the physician's knowledge and experience jointly with coarse data about the patient's present health state and clinical history, without further ado. This kind of prognosis is justified for simple cases, such as the common cold, which are the vast majority seen by family doctors.

In the olden days, the clinical method consisted in listening to the patient's complaints and performing a cursory clinical examination. Nowadays, the internal medicine practitioner will want to see, in addition, the results of some laboratory tests, for he seeks to frame a prognosis based on a diagnosis involving hypotheses about both the pathogenic mechanisms and the mechanisms of action of the treatment he envisages. By acting in this way, the modern doctor puts into practice the praxiological rule "Learn before acting" and, more specifically, the scientistic one, "To plan a course of action, such as a medical protocol, use the best available knowledge." Obviously, this rule contravenes the pragmatist philosophy.

This procedure is far superior to the traditional one but, of course, it is not error-free. A common source of error is missing a key variable, as a consequence of which the corresponding biomarker has not been checked. Another source of error is that, either because of a mutation or because of a delayed effect of an earlier sickness, the patient suffers from an "idiopathy" so ill defined and uncommon that the physician has never met it before. When a medical prognosis goes wrong, the rationalist will attempt to find the error sources, in an effort to learn. The mystic, by contrast, may interpret the unexpected recovery as a miracle performed by a saintly deceased. This is how many a sainthood has been awarded.

Whatever the error source in diagnosis or prognosis, it can be minimized by combining the clinical approach with the statistical one, which we first met in Section 4.2. The *mechanical* or *algorithmic* method enriches the same clinical data about the individual patient with statistical data and algorithms. These data are statements of the form "$f\%$ of D patients of sex S and age A, treated with therapy T, recovered in so many days." If the patient fits a box like this, his physician will be able to make a decision supported by a pile of well-documented cases — unless of course the patient suffers from an idiopathy.

As we saw in Section 4.2, the merits and shortcomings of the two methods were vehemently discussed in the mid-twentieth century. As was to be expected, the sympathizers of the "soft" philosophies and pseudo-philosophies favored the traditional or clinical approach, whereas the partisans of scientism supported the statistical one. As it usually happens in such cases, more heat than light was generated, until the clinical psychologist and philosopher of science Paul Meehl (1954) asked and investigated the only relevant question: which of the two methods predicts better? Meehl's answer was unequivocal: the statistical predictions are more exact than the clinical ones. Ulterior investigations (e.g., Grove *et al.* 2000: 25) confirmed and refined Meehl's conclusion.

This finding did not surprise those familiar with the research of Daniel Kahneman (2011) and his school (Kahneman *et al.* 1982). They investigated intuitive reasoning, that is, spontaneous and fast reasoning in contrast to deductive argument, which is algorithmic or subject to rule. In particular, they investigated the traps into which fast reasoning can fall. In medicine, the most common fallacy is "Disease D is manifested as syndrome S. Now, subject b exhibits syndrome S. Ergo, b suffers from D." Another common medical fallacy before the advent of controlled trials was *post hoc, ergo propter hoc* ("after this, because of this"). This fallacy was no less than the rationale for carefully noting and keeping case histories — the only source of medical knowledge until the birth of experimental medicine in the mid-nineteenth century.

Another dangerous cognitive trap is that, as Francis Bacon (1905: 780) noted four centuries ago, we tend to count our hits but not our misses. The research by Einhorn and Hogarth (1978) confirmed that insight: clinicians tend to overestimate their evaluations, so they do not ask for feedback, and miss the opportunity to correct their bad mental habits. The moral is clear: since algorithmic reasoning is less uncertain and expensive than intuitive reasoning, mechanize as far as possible. That is, let us realize Leibniz's dream of replacing inconclusive verbal disputation with computation. With one proviso, though: computation is reliable because it is not creative. Hence, it must be used to work out and implement original ideas, not to replace them.

At the other end of the opinions spectrum, we find the preference for empirical indicators over evidence-based medicine, the way Hayward and Krumholz (2012) did when evaluating the standard cholesterol-control therapy. The key to improving scientific prognosis is not to go back to empiricism, but to combine medical statistics with the biology of the pathogeny and the pharmacodynamics of the drugs. This combination is all the more to be preferred because mechanical prognosis cannot embrace all the possible relevant variables.

Finally, let us warn once again against the abuse of the term 'probability.' The "mechanical" (or statistical) method does not allow us to make statements of the form "The recovery probability is p," because it relies on statistics and actuarial tables, which include frequencies. Frequencies are collective or mass properties, whereas probabilities are predicated of individual states or events; furthermore, the frequency concept is empirical, whereas that of probability is theoretical. Hence, serious talk of probabilities is only possible in connection with probabilistic theories. And so far, these have not been found in medicine, because this discipline deals with causal processes, not random ones.

8.2 Individual and Collective Prevention

"An ounce of prevention is worth a pound of cure." This wise old principle, part of the Hippocratic teaching, was updated in recent times by requiring that every action that might harm health or the environment be endorsed by the relevant scientific studies — for instance, by randomized controlled trials in the case of therapies, and by epidemiological research in that of social policies. This modern version of commonsensical prudence is known as the *precautionary principle*.

Since ancient times, all good medics have abided by that principle, since they have not only striven to cure their patients, but also to keep them well. The main preventive measures have always been diet, cleanliness, physical activity, and moderation in everything. From time to time, further preventive panaceas have been widely adopted. One of them, cod liver oil, was claimed to protect from colds and cut the risk of the most common non-communicable ailments, from diabetes and cardiovascular disease to cancer — without any hard evidence (Rizos *et al.* 2012). The same holds for vitamin C megadosis, antioxidants, and "probiotic" food. From the *Cochrane Reviews*, we learn that none of the three most popular medications to prevent the common cold — garlic, vitamin C, and zinc — works to that effect, though the last two have a modest effect in reducing the duration of the disease.

Doctors can and do recommend certain behaviors to keep in good health, but they cannot accomplish much with bad patients — those who either do not listen to good advice or cannot afford them. This is why much of a physician's job is "firefighting." Since exhortations to change unhealthy behaviors are often ineffectual, preventive medicine must target mainly "automatic processes," i.e., those triggered by environmental stimuli, such as commercial ads and availability of unhealthy food. But to control environmental health hazards, we must start by identifying them, a task that has only begun. Here are a few examples.

1) We have only recently learned that fast food — the staple of the over-worked urban citizen and the uncontrolled teenager with pocket money — is bad for you if only because of its excess in three harmful and strongly addictive ingredients — fat, salt, and sugar. Nobody knows whether radical changes in diet, such as those caused by the Neolithic Revolution, prolonged famines, and the current fast food fad, are accompanied by genetic changes. But we do know what happened to the genomes of wolves when they got domesticated, and thus changed from carnivores into herbivores: they increased the number of genes for amylase, an enzyme critical for digesting starch. Will our remote descendants acquire *Mc* genes?

2) As recently as around 1950, it was learned that cigarette smoking not only harms the cardiovascular system, but also causes lung cancer. It took several decades of fierce political fight to force the powerful tobacco industry to label their products as dangerous to health. By contrast, the battle for gun control has barely begun as I write, and it won't be won unless the U.S. government sets the example, by stopping torture, capital punishment, and militarism.

3) Many carcinogenic agents, such as pesticides, herbicides, high-energy radiation, and certain food components, are man-made, hence in principle susceptible to strict controls. But they are also important revenue

sources, so that their control in the interest of public health would conflict with certain business interests. An obvious example is the clash between "organic" farming and agrobusiness — a conflict that is yet to be resolved, and in any case lies beyond the reach of individual medics. This is where local politics and non-governmental organizations can trigger important changes. Just think of "greening" school and hospital lunches, and protecting "organic" agricultural cooperatives.

To make things worse, influential medicine critics, like Iván Illich, Thomas Szasz, and Michel Foucault, have accused it of causing diseases. The truth is that, while comparatively few treatments are harmful, infectious diseases spread easily in hospitals and other health care facilities. For example, in the USA alone, about 100,000 people die annually due to infections acquired there. But this only suggests that the current preventive practices are inadequate. This problem is so serious and so complex, that it should be tackled by an interdisciplinary team of microbiologists, epidemiologists, management experts, and architects.

The enemies of medicine have also attacked medical prevention, claiming that annual checkups are unnecessary when not harmful, that they are just an aspect of the "medicalization" of society — the attempt to pass off social issues as medical problems. Even Petr Skrabanek (2000), habitually an intelligent commentator on the state of medicine, objected to giving advice on lifestyles, and went so far as to call *health fascism* the coercive measures governments take to protect public health, such as banning smoking in public places and selling alcohol to minors.

All physicians know that poor diet, obesity, alcoholism, smoking, uncleanliness, inactivity, and unsafe sex kill millions of people every year. The Framingham Heart Study (1948 to today), which initially involved 5,000 people in Framingham, Massachusetts, exhibited the main risk factors for cardiovascular and related diseases: all of them, particularly smoking, alcoholism, and poor diet, are lifestyle-related. The Canadian INTERHEART Study on myocardial infarction, conducted on 29,000 individuals in 52 countries, confirmed and extended the results of the Framingham Study, showing that 90% of this risk is preventable. These studies also suggest why women outlive men: they smoke and drink less;

why the Chinese have a low rate of cardiovascular disease: their diet is vegetable-intensive; and why Canadians have healthier hearts than Americans: they exercise more.

Think also that, since falls are the main cause of injury in older adults, physiotherapists can do much to prevent such accidents by teaching seniors to relearn to walk, turn around, sit up, get up, and shower safely. A single session with a physiotherapist can teach all this, decreasing by 30% the frequency of falls. Regrettably, sports medicine, bodybuilding, and studying the gait of racehorses have been more fashionable and lucrative than helping the fragile elderly to move around.

The critics of preventive medicine, none of whom has made any original contributions to the social sciences, have not understood that unhealthy habits, from sedentarism to fast-food eating, to smoking to alcoholism to sexual promiscuity, are social issues as well as medical problems, so that they should be tackled from both sides. Far from proposing solutions to the social question, those authors are part of it since, in the wake of Nietzsche, they debase science, morals, progressive social reforms — particularly in the public health domain — and even rationality. Their writings constitute thus a health hazard in addition to a political one. Fortunately, they have not discouraged the WHO or the local sanitary authorities from taking a number of preventive measures, from vaccination and drinking-water purification and fluoridation to comprehensive tobacco, alcohol, salt, and trans fats controls through taxation. The dramatic gains in health brought about by such policies around the world are well known (e.g., Ezzati & Riboli 2012). It is less well known that clinical intervention — individual medicine — is a very small fraction of preventive medicine (e.g., Shelton 2013).

The North Karelia Project, one of the most sensational and successful social experiments ever, proved that a systemic approach with strong grassroots can improve dramatically, in a short time and at a low cost, the lifestyles and lifespans of a whole community (McAlistair *et al.* 1981). This government project, started in 1972, was conceived and directed by the physician Pekka Puska, and was strongly supported by the Martha Organization, a housewives group. The program involved persuading people to adopt a low-fat and low-salt diet rich in vegetables and fruits, as well as to quit smoking. The results of these changes were an 82% decline in cardiovascular disease, and a 7% rise in the life expectancy of men — all these in less than a decade. The moral seems obvious:

Preventive public health policy + Popular participation = Public health gain.

The epidemics that have ravaged humankind since the Neolithic Era should have taught us millennia ago that health should concern us all, instead of being treated as a private good. Only hermits have the right to catch preventable diseases; the rest of us have the duty to keep well, not only for our own sake but also for that of our neighbors, as well as to avoid becoming public burdens.

Social medicine, which focuses on the social conditions relevant to health, was born in Western Europe at the end of the nineteenth century. Initially, it was a social movement — called 'social hygiene' — led by physicians, public servants, and politicians. Its central goal was to prod governments to design and implement inclusive and vast public health policies, from sanitary infrastructure to universal health coverage. The European Left participated in this movement as a progressive social reform. And the most enlightened custodians of the British, German, and Austrian Empires, from Bismarck to Churchill, supported public health care both to take the wind out of the sails of social democracy, and to strengthen their armed forces, who had no use for recruits as weak and sick as the members of the general population (Gilbert 1966).

Recently, the same motive impelled a group of retired officers of the American armed forces to declare that the current epidemics of child obesity constitutes a national security hazard, as overweight individuals are health risks and bad combatants. (Being overweight is defined as having a body mass index greater than 30 kilograms/square meters, and the optimal value for longevity is $25\,kg/m^2$.) Yet, today's conservative politicians — who would have been called 'reactionaries' only one generation ago — do not understand that health and security go hand in hand. Nor do they understand that prevention is the key to cost control and improving the quality of health care (Emanuel 2012).

Public health has ancient roots, the most striking being the Roman aqueducts and sewers, as well as the ban on burying the dead inside the city walls, the cleanup of mosquito-infested swamps, and the use of quarantine to contain epidemics. Rome started to build its extensive network of underground sewers in the sixth century B.C., and part of its monumental *Cloaca maxima* is still in use. In addition, there were public baths and latrines at every Roman military camp. (By contrast, the Italian soldiers in the First World War had to defecate in the open, which is why more of them died from dysentery and related infections than from bullet wounds.) The admirable Roman sanitary system was the work of civil servants, military officers, engineers, craftsmen, and slave laborers. Their accomplishments were all the more remarkable given the backwardness of Roman medics compared to their Greek teachers (Sigerist 1883).

The ancient Roman state paid the salaries of the medics who assisted the poor, and it maintained public hospitals besides the military hospitals spread throughout the Empire. It also founded and maintained the earliest public medical schools. But the Roman surgeons worked without knowing much anatomy; they confined themselves to stitching and cauterizing flesh wounds, setting bones, and amputating limbs. They could hardly do more, since anatomy was born only in the sixteenth century. In any case, the Roman statesmen knew something that many of our politicians refuse to learn: that in a civilized society, public health is a central concern of government at all levels.

Nowadays, every developed nation has a ministry of public health, and since 1948, one of the main components of the United Nations is the WHO, in charge of forecasting, preventing, and managing global epidemics. True, this organization is too heavy and it has made some serious errors, such as promoting "alternative medicines" and wildly exaggerating the magnitude of the previous flu pandemic. But these are reasons for demanding the reform of the WHO, not for destroying it.

Let us briefly recall the nature and role of epidemiology, an essential tool of public health policy-making. The main task of epidemiologists is to look for statistical associations among variables of medical interest, in hopes of finding underlying causal relations. This is how it was finally proved that smoking causes lung cancer, and that excess sugar ingestion predisposes to diabetes mellitus. But for every good epidemiological study, there is at least one bad one. Thus, a few years ago, it was reported that cabbage kills cancer cells — provided it is used in combination with chemotherapy.

The vagaries of epidemiology led Petr Skrabanek (2000: 144) to writing that "there is an epidemic of epidemiologists." Such destructive criticism is irresponsible and contrary to the tradition of constructive criticism prevalent in the scientific community. But of course, the search for statistical correlations among variables picked at random should be discouraged; only properties suspected of being involved in mechanisms of action are worth being studied.

For instance, it makes sense to investigate the correlation between scholastic achievement and parasitosis, because intestinal parasites weaken. But it would be foolish to study the correlation between political orientation and cancer, because the former does not exist at the molecular level.

In addition to studying the social context of disease, an epidemiologist may design public health policies; he may do sanitary engineering and, acting in this capacity, he may warn or advise the public, and engage with public health authorities. It suffices to mention two topical sociomedical problems: those of drug addiction and obesity. Everyone, save for some religious fanatics and political demagogues, knows that the so-called War on Drugs is being won by the drug cartels, because the sale of narcotics is the most profitable business as long as it remains in criminal hands. Contrary to what some political philosophers have claimed, the uncontrolled market is a school of vice, not virtue.

All the experts have been saying for decades that the only solution to the drug problem is to legalize the consumption of narcotics while strictly controlling their sales, the way it is done in several European nations. It is also well known that the "war on bulge" can best be "fought" by combining dietetic education with the expansion of physical education in schools and a stiff tax on sugar. (Taxation is the only known method to reduce demand.) In sum, epidemiologists can make capital contributions to governance. (For the impact of the biosocial and social sciences and technologies on governance, see Bunge 2009.)

However, in political democracies, voters and advocacy groups are major contributors to the design of health care policies. Since about 1990, more than 1,000 American organizations advocating the interests of patients of special diseases, such as AIDS and breast cancer, have acquired significant political clout, and have secured extra funding for research on those diseases. Although this sectoral approach (one advocacy group per disease) may yield short-term benefits, it is likely to be harmful in the long run, because it politicizes and balkanizes biomedical research; it punishes research on other severe ailments (such as prostate cancer and arthritis); and it shifts health policy-making from scientists to activists.

Let us now glance at another biosocial science: demography. It is well known that, in the prosperous nations, life expectancy at birth has doubled between 1850 and 1950. The vulgar opinion is that this sensational achievement is due to medical advances. The physician and demographer Thomas McKeown (1967) and his school challenged this opinion: they held that the rapid improvement in health was mainly due to better nutrition and to sanitary works, especially sewers and water purification, combined with compulsory vaccination and city planning. In short, *corpore sano in civitas sana*.

The *McKeown thesis*, as it is usually called, was corrected on minor points, but its central message has been confirmed: the natural and social surroundings as well as the social conditions — especially employment, housing, education, and access to public health care — are critical determinants of health, hence of longevity (see Stuckler & Siegler 2011). This finding corroborated the thesis of the social hygiene movement, around 1900, that health improves with sanitation and the standard of living.

The most recent review of the social determinants of health in Europe (Marmot *et al.* 2012) confirms the thesis that "[s]ocially cohesive societies, which are increasingly affluent, with developed welfare states and high-quality education and health services," have resulted in "remarkable health gains," some of which have been lost since the onset of the economic slump that started in 2008. In short, the evidence has vindicated McKeown's thesis.

Contrary to what the enemies of public health care assert, the McKeown thesis does not propose *replacing* personal responsibility for one's lifestyle with socialized medicine; it only urges facilitating the implementation of personal decisions. For instance, the best of intentions about sanitary housing, healthy nutrition, and regular medical checkups cannot be realized without the requisite wherewithal. American medicine may well be the most advanced in the world, but the Scandinavians, Dutch, British, Australians, New Zealanders, and Germans get better health care — and at half the price.

Public health care and education are some of the first victims of economic recessions, political right-turns, and uncontrolled social explosions. The recent history of syphilis in China is a case in point. As soon as they seized power, the Chinese communists attacked syphilis, and all but eradicated it within a few years. But this scourge re-emerged four decades later along with the country's swift modernization, and has kept growing almost exponentially ever since. The process has been roughly like this:

$\uparrow$ *Social inequality* $\rightarrow$ *Rural exodus & sexual freedom* $\rightarrow$ $\uparrow$ *Prostitution* $\rightarrow$ $\uparrow$ *Syphilis.*

(Notice that the source of this process is income *inequality*, rather than absolute *poverty*. When everyone is poor, no one complains. In society, as in nature, forces are generated by gradients. If the economists who designed the World Bank had known this, that organization's mission would have been the decrease in income inequality rather than the eradication of poverty.)

In another case relevant to the McKeown thesis, the South African government recently reversed its previous stand about the AIDS epidemic; it admitted its reality and started a massive medical treatment of the population to cure AIDS victims and stop the propagation of the HIV. No doubt, this decision was correct, but it did not work as well as intended because it was sectoral rather than systemic; it ignored the old Roman maxim, *Leges sine moribus vanae* ("Laws without customs are void"). In fact, the AIDS problem is sociomedical rather than purely medical; it involves ignorance, in particular the superstitions fomented by the practitioners of aboriginal medicine; the opposition of the Catholic Church to the use of condoms; and the sexual promiscuity associated with macho pride.

The preceding refers to the practical or normative branch of social medicine. This is a *biosocial technology* because, to attain certain practical ends, it uses some medical findings along with others derived from the study and management of society. The descriptive branch of social medicine is descriptive epidemiology. This is a basic biosocial science, as are demography, anthropology, and psychology.

The sheer existence of biosocial science confutes the basic dogma of the hermeneutic (or "interpretive") approach that the social and the natural sciences do not intersect — as if psychology, demography, and epidemiology did not exist. This dogma is not an isolated piece but an essential component of hermeneutic anthropology, according to which everything human would be basically spiritual or symbolic, and the latter immaterial, hence alien to the sciences of matter (Dilthey 1883).

This idealist philosophy has exerted a strong influence on the social studies, in shifting attention from work and artifacts to symbols and ceremonies, from statistics to legends, and from reason to intuition (see Bunge 1996a, 1998b). Hermeneutics holds that social life is a text or narrative that must be interpreted or deciphered rather than explained, but it does not supply interpretation rules, so that it is impossible to know whether one narrative is truer than another. This school, very visible in the humanities, has hardly affected medical practice.

So far, the influence of hermeneutics on medicine has been confined to confusing disease with diagnosis, and to overrating the importance of the clinical history. This exaggeration bears the name of *narrative medicine* (Charon 2006). Its practitioners promise to improve medical diagnosis and assistance through persuading medics to listen more carefully to what their patients tell them, learning to empathize with them, improving the literary quality of their clinical histories, and even writing "parallel histories" recording what the doctor feels while treating his patients. There are no trials to check the professional competence of the graduates of the narrative medicine program at Columbia University. Back to epidemiology, born two centuries before philosophical hermeneutics.

The mere existence of epidemiology also ruins two reductionist programs: *biologism*, the branch of naturalism according to which everything social is basically biological; and *sociologism*, which claims that medicine is a social science. Biologism, in particular the attempt to explain everything social in genetic or evolutionary terms, ignores the fact that the rules of social behavior are invented, corrected, and abandoned, and that not all of them are adaptive. (Just think of war, slavery, justice as revenge, the death penalty, ethnic cleansing, bans on planned parenthood, and honor killing.) As for sociologism, it cannot even account for the differences between sex and marriage, occasional violence and organized crime, or biological groups and formal organizations — let alone between biological evolution and human history.

Reduction should be sought and welcomed when it explains correctly, as in the case of the study of genetic and degenerative diseases, as well as in the study of the stunting of biological and cognitive development as an effect of extreme poverty. But reduction impoverishes when the facts themselves are hybrid, as is the case with contagion, stress, child abuse, rape, and food riots. When a fact happens at the intersection of two different levels of organization, a *multidisciplinary* approach — a particular case of the systemic approach — is apposite.

This approach is adopted tacitly by contemporary medicine (recall Section 2.3). Regrettably, systemism is often mistaken for holism, and most students of society and social philosophers are still attached to philosophical individualism, despite the fact that it denies the existence of the very object of *social* science, which is not the individual but social systems, from band to family to gang to business firm to state and nation (see Bunge 1979; Wan 2011).

Individualism is not only at variance with social reality; it is also a health hazard, as it rejects the very ideas of a sanitary system, compulsory vaccination, and epidemics management. For example, the U.S. Centers for Disease Control and Prevention have recently issued an alert to the "baby boomers," for many of them unknowingly carry the hepatitis C virus, which calls for medical treatment and is contagious. State interference of this kind is opposed by the "libertarian" ideology hatched by such radical individualists as Herbert Spencer, Frederick Hayek, Milton Friedman, and Ayn Rand. According to them, everyone should be allowed to "do their own thing" without government interference. But in health matters, there is no such thing as doing one's own thing, both because everyone is a walking germ bomb, and because every normal person feels the duty to help others.

In short, universal health care can do much to prevent disease. However, since most diseases have many causes, we should not run toward the mirage of a single preventive measure; health care is multifaceted, hence it calls for the systemic approach that inheres in systemic materialism.

8.3 Longevity at All Costs?

Life expectancy at birth has doubled or tripled since about 1800 in all prosperous nations. Even in China, where Western medicine is still a rarity, it doubled in the course of the last century — a striking evidence in support of McKeown's socioeconomic approach to health care.

However, this achievement is double-edged. Undoubtedly, it is nice to live as long as one enjoys the ride. But aging increases the risk of falling prey to diseases that kill the joy of living, such as arthritis, Parkinson's disease, and steep cognitive decay. Besides, in the advanced nations, the elderly tend to consume up to two-thirds of the health care budget. So, it is not worth pursuing ripe old age for its own sake; only an enjoyable and productive old age is to be sought.

The remarkable increase in life expectancy has revived the age-old illusion of immortality. Thus, the cover of *Time* magazine for February 21, 2011, announced: "2045: The Year Man Becomes Immortal." Who could reasonably believe this extraordinary prophecy? Obviously, it is untestable at best because, even supposing that no one were to die after 2045, we would have to wait an eternity to be sure.

In any event, gerontologists do not adopt the empiricist attitude of standing by and watching; they study the aging mechanisms, and have learned that, although they can be slowed down, the end of life cannot be staved off indefinitely. And the vast majority of us do not devote our lives to learning the *ars moriendi*, but to living as best we can. As the priest in the classic film *Roma città aperta* declares as he is about to be shot by the fascists, "What is hard is not to die well but to live well."

Some of the most important recent gerontological research concerns the impact of caloric restriction on both healthspan and lifespan. Until recently, it was widely believed, on the strength of studies conducted on rodents, that eating 10%–40% less significantly prolongs life because it improves health. The latest randomized controlled trial of this kind was conducted on rhesus monkeys, comparatively long-lived animals (Mattison *et al.* 2012). This study, begun in 1987 at the National Institute of Health Animal Center, has unequivocally shown that, while caloric restriction does indeed lower morbidity, it does not affect longevity. This finding was unexpected and so far unexplained. The 16 authors of this study concluded by stating that it will be valuable "to dissect the mechanisms behind the improvement in health that occurred with and without significant effects on survival."

The astonishing finding that lifespan is independent of caloric intake holds an important lesson for those of us who can and will do something about our own lifestyle. We used to believe that the reward for clean and austere living was a long life. Now, we learn that the reward for cleanliness and frugality is a healthy life. In light of this finding, we should also revise the traditional rule of medical ethics, that enjoins physicians to prolong life at all costs. Indeed, the said clinical trial suggests maximizing healthspan rather than lifespan, which in turn confirms the humanist maxim, *Enjoy life and help live.*

Coda

Health care professionals have practiced preventive medicine whenever they have given prophylactic and dietetic advice. However, large-scale preventive medicine started two millennia before the birth of modern medicine, namely when the ancient Romans began building sewers, aqueducts, and pipes for the home delivery of drinking water. This task was interrupted during the Middle Ages, and resumed in the nineteenth century in Western Europe and some of its dependencies, where the public sanitary works were combined with massive vaccination and, among the educated, with periodic checkups. As argued in Section 8.2, those large-scale measures, more than the great therapeutic advances, have prolonged lifespan.

Yet, some religious and political groups, as well as advocates of CAMs (complementary and alternative medicines), are still campaigning against compulsory vaccination. This campaign was reinforced by an article by an obscure surgeon published in 1998 by the prestigious *Lancet* — but since retracted — who claimed, without any evidence, that the MMR vaccine (for diphtheria, whooping cough, and tetanus) causes autism. This harmful piece of "news" spread quickly because it appeared in a prestigious medical periodical, and because of the mistrust that science inspires among the semi-educated (see Goldacre 2010: Chapter 12). Back to the increase in lifespan.

Longevity has increased so much that it has revived the myth of eternal life. George Bernard Shaw made it the subject of his famous comedy *Back* to *Methuselah* (1921). This myth resurfaces once in a while in books that promise immortality *through not dying*, as Woody Allen proclaimed confidently in one of his movies moments before facing a firing squad. All adults know that they must eventually die.

But the idea of immortality raises the interesting philosophical problem of whether it is possible to *prove* that "All men are mortal" is more than just an inductive generalization. A consistent empiricist will argue that, since the generalization in question was born as an induction, it must remain that, so that we should not rule out the possibility that an immortal human being will be born some day. A gerontologist, by contrast, will argue that the various aging mechanisms start working as soon as youth ends: programmed cellular death, shortening of telomeres, accumulation of heavy metals and toxins, increase in the areas of scar tissue, decreasing muscle mass, and so on. Consequently, the proposition "All men are mortal" has ceased to be a mere empirical generalization, to become a genuine scientific law. We have also learned that theologians and poets have overrated death, for there is neither beauty nor nobility in it — death is just the termination of life.

To live an enjoyable, long, and productive life, there is nothing better than to live a clean life in a clean environment; to engage in activities that bring social recognition; and to abstain from the whimpering typical of Romantic poets and existentialist scribblers. To minimize suffering and mess, one should attempt to die suddenly and in good health — from heart failure or massive stroke. But, for better or for worse, we cannot choose either end. As for the survivors, the humanists enjoin them to stop the fuss, help clean up the mess, and support the grieving.

Of course, periodic medical checkups help lengthen the lifespan, if only for the early detection of life-threatening processes. However, beware of overdiagnosis: some doctors prescribe too many tests, to make sure that their diagnoses are correct, and that nothing may go wrong with their patients in the far future. But all invasive tests and all radical medications take their toll, and some of them may unwittingly cause diseases, as Welch *et al.* (2011) have argued. In short, the pursuit of certainty may be as bad as total ignorance, in health matters as in all others. Moderate skepticism counsels moderation in everything but love: you can never love enough or be loved enough.

CHAPTER 9

IATROETHICS

9.1 Ethical Schools

Human behavior is subject not only to natural laws but also to rules — which is why biologism does not work. Humans invent, adopt, alter, or repeal rules of two types: legal and moral. Whereas the former change with social structure, moral norms, though also not engraved in the genes, change more slowly. This is because morality fits not only interests and reasons — most of which are circumstantial — but also the social emotions, such as empathy and sympathy, as well as the need to live together with others. Such co-living (*convivencia*) would be impossible without a modicum of honesty, altruism, and readiness to resolve conflicts.

Physicians are subject not only to the legal norms intended to regulate the behavior of all citizens, but also to special moral rules adapted to their primary goal: to treat the ailing. Some of these rules are "Do not invent diseases," "Do not prescribe treatments known to be either ineffective or harmful," "Try to keep abreast of medical progress," and "Offer medical assistance even without a guarantee that it will be remunerated." True, some members of the medical profession occasionally break this or that rule of the medical code. But such deviations are exceptional and, when made known, they hurt the reputation of the transgressors, and may even cause sanctions.

Medical praxis, unlike shamanism, has been regulated in all civilizations. But medical ethics, or iatroethics, seem to have emerged explicitly only with the Hippocratic Oath, perhaps the earliest secular and voluntary moral code. Although it is usually said that the top principle of this foundational document is "Do no harm," it also mandated active assistance of the sick, whether free or enslaved (*Epidemics* I, XI). In fact, the members of the Cos school also practiced surgery; for example, they removed stones from gall bladders. But it is true that, contrary to the Ayurvedic medics, who earned a reputation for their surgical dexterity and audacity, the Hippocratics were cautious.

Medical ethics has undergone many changes since the mid-nineteenth century. Some new moral problems have emerged, such as what to do with patients in prolonged coma, and problems that used to be kept secret, such as those referring to sex and reproduction, are now being openly debated (e.g., Veatch 1997). Moreover, starting in the 1960s, bioethics has attracted a large number of practitioners — initially amateurs, as in all new fields — and is often wedded to science's traditional enemy — religion. Unsurprisingly, religious bioethics enjoy the support of conservative politicians and wealthy think tanks and foundations.

However, nowadays, most bioethical problems tend to be discussed outside the narrow boxes of the authoritarian ethical doctrines anchored to religions. Just think of the free sale of contraceptives, abortion on demand, assisted death, embryonic stem cell research, the taking of narcotics under medical supervision, and the forcible confinement of pathogen carriers. Or think of the expansion of universal health care, the criminalization of large-scale pollution, and the ethical restrictions on medical experimentation ruled by the Nuremberg Code.

In this chapter, we shall glance at only a minute fraction of the issues discussed in the vast contemporary bioethical literature. However, contrary to the standard bioethical discussions, we shall start by postulating some general ethical principles, since ethics is supposed to be principled rather than opportunistic, as well as part of philosophy — hence a discipline with logical, ontological, and epistemological commitments — rather than an autonomous discipline. Let us start by recalling the main current ethical concerns.

1) *Amoralism*: good and evil are fictitious rather than objective, and consequently, moral rules are just social conventions, when not ruses to fool people. This is roughly the view advanced by Nietzsche in his *Beyond Good and Evil* (1886). Sometimes he interchanged 'amoralism' and 'immoralism.'

2) *Immoralism* or *nihilism*: we have no obligations except to ourselves. Thus spoke the pop philosopher Ayn Rand, a defender of "rational

egoism" and an idol of the American far right. It was also the slogan of the Italian fascist militia: *Me ne frego* ("I could not care less" in polite translation).

3) *Radical individualism* (Nietzsche's amoralism, Ayn Rand's rational egoism, and the Tea Party's libertarianism): "There is no such thing as society: there are only individuals" (Margaret Thatcher). This doctrine not only denies the existence of impersonal values and the need for morals; it is also impractical, because no one can survive without help from others, and because antisocial behavior is usually reprimanded or even punished.

4) *Holism*: "You are nothing: Your *Volk* [people, nation, ethnic community] is everything" (Nazi slogan); "Everything inside the state, nothing outside the state, nobody against the state" (Benito Mussolini); "Good is only that which favors the Party" (Vladimir Ilich Lenin).

5) *Negative utilitarianism*: Do no harm (*Primum non nocere*). This was the view of Buddha, Hippocrates, and Popper. It is insufficient, for coexistence in any social group calls for mutual help. It is also impracticable, because many interventions, from education to surgery to quarantine to incarceration involve causing pain.

6) *Religious ethics* attempt to subordinate morals to ancient dogmas and practices at variance with science. They concern only the duties (never the rights) of the members of a religious congregation, and their precepts are taken to be eternal and above debate. Almost all religious ethics are local, circumstantial, and obsolete. The monotheistic ethics are totalitarian, in the sense that they cover all the aspects of life, from sex to property to dealings with fellow members of the congregation (to be helped), as well as with aliens (to be distrusted). No religious ethics, except for the Quaker one, admits human rights or defends any of the modern social values — liberty, equality, solidarity, democracy, tolerance, peace, social justice, or free inquiry. This is why no important progressive political movement has ever adopted any religious ethics. For the same reason, biomedical researchers do not abide by them, as became clear in recent years in relation to policies on stem cell research and reproduction. The U.S. President's Council on Bioethics, set up by Bill Clinton, and which

under George W. Bush had become a right-wing think tank, was dissolved by Barack Obama.

7) *Deontology*: "Do your duties." This moral philosophy, Confucius' and Kant's, is the secular version of religious ethics. It is universalist (rather than tribal or sectarian), but it does not tell us which are our duties, who is to specify them, nor whether we earn any rights in exchange for behaving dutifully; it is the good servant's morality. This is why Kant's deontology is not included in any pro-democracy political philosophy. Unsurprisingly, Confucianism is politically docile, and Kant opposed democracy.

8) *Contractualism*: "Being moral is keeping contracts." This legalistic doctrine — held in various forms by Thomas Hobbes, Jean-Jacques Rousseau, and John Rawls — disregards the facts that not all agreements are fair, and that children and the disempowered are in no position to sign on the dotted line. Nor does it apply to those who, like the Doctors Without Borders volunteers, risk their lives without expecting any external rewards.

9) *Utilitarianism*: "Strive to maximize your own expected utility (individualist utilitarianism) or that of the greatest number (social utilitarianism)." Standard medical ethics is utilitarian, in that it enjoins physicians to maximize lifespan regardless of the quality of life. However, utilitarianism is open to several objections. First, spontaneous or non-calculated actions, as well as altruistic ones, escape the utilitarian calculus. Second, the very notion of expected utility is problematic, as it combines the notions of subjective utility and subjective probability, neither of which is well defined (Bunge 1996a).

10) *Humanism* or *agathonism*: egotuism, or a combination of egoism with altruism. Top principle: *Enjoy life and help live* (Bunge 1989).

The ethics traditionally taught in medical schools is usually called 'deontology.' Actually, it is broader than the Kantian ethics, for it emphasizes professional competence and it includes the precautionary principle as well as the need to secure the patient's informed consent. The rights of patients have also been added in recent times, in contrast to traditional medical paternalism.

Let us see next how the above-mentioned general principles fare in both medical practice and health care policy-making.

9.2 Individual Medical Ethics

I submit that secular humanism is the only one of the 10 major ethical schools that entrenches the rights and duties of the individual recognized in the most advanced modern societies. Moreover, humanism is the only one that defines "justice" as the balance of rights (or freedoms) with duties (or burdens). What follows should confirm this view. In fact, the application of humanism to medical practice involves the following special norms:

N1 Autonomy: Every conscious human being is the only rightful owner of his/her own body.

N2 Everyone has the moral right to medical assistance.

N3 Everyone has the moral obligation of caring for his/her own health and that of his/her neighbors, as well as of keeping his/her surroundings in a good sanitary state.

N4 Health workers ought to treat patients using only therapies approved by state-of-the-art biomedical research within their reach.

N5 All health workers should seek to observe William Osler's maxim: *Absolute safety and full consent.*

N6 Medics ought to protect their patients from the demands of political, religious, or medical sects that put their health at risk.

N7 Health workers have the right to join professional unions and protect themselves from unfair medical malpractice accusations, but they also have the duty to ensure basic health care services at all times.

The preceding norms, together with the maximal principle concerning the right to enjoy life and the duty to help others do the same, constitute a conceptual *system* rather than a haphazard collection of statements. Yet, when applied to individual cases, some of them may enter into conflict with others, and the application of any one of them may require the simultaneous application of others. For example, the right to health care does not give anyone the right to hoard scarce medicaments or medical services. Let us now glance at some of the consequences of the preceding norms.

Here are some consequences of Norm 1 ("I own myself."): (a) children are not owned by their parents or by the state, and women are not owned by their husbands or bosses; (b) the right to love comes together with the obligation to provide for the offspring; (c) slavery, torture, child abuse, "honor" killings, and rape are immoral; (d) capital punishment is inadmissible: legal murder is still murder; (e) suicide and assisted death are rightful as long as the deceased does not leave impecunious dependents; (f) women are responsible for their own reproductive health; and (g) the state has the right to control the birth rate when sustainability is at risk.

The same Norm 1, about the autonomy of the person, confers sexual freedom but not sexual promiscuity, which puts health and family at risk. More importantly, we should be able to resort to Norm 1 to defend ourselves from the corporations that are patenting our genes as if they, rather than evolution, had created them (Koepsell 2009). Note, incidentally, that the "pro-life" crusaders do not object to this usurpation — nor to capital punishment, "honor crimes," "enhanced interrogation techniques" (torture), rape, and other encroachments on the autonomy of the person.

Norm 2 (right to health care) implies that, unless all citizens can afford to join effective mutual help associations, the state has the obligation to offer free and competent health care — as in fact it is doing so in nearly all the developed nations. However, when the public health care facilities become overloaded, governments should be able to make deals with private clinics, to ensure that no sick individuals wait in long lines.

Norm 3 (personal health and environment) has a solid medical ground: those who neglect their own health endanger other people's; much the same holds for those who foul their surroundings. Besides, the offenders of both kinds strain the commonwealth's resources.

However, Norm 3 should be qualified: (a) medics are expected to be *concerned* about their patients but not to get personally *involved* with them; they should stay at arm's length from them in order to preserve their own objectivity, rationality, and calm; and (b) medics should be able to refuse treating individuals who endanger their safety or that of their staff.

Norm 4 (competent medical practice) is intended to keep the population in good health, in particular to protect it from medical quackery. But, since high-quality medical resources are becoming increasingly scarce and expensive, there is the danger that medical assistance will mirror the increasing income inequalities among regions and among individuals. The Netherlands, Scandinavia, the UK, Australia, Canada, and a few other nations have avoided this elitization of health care by keeping a "single tier" or egalitarian medical assistance managed by the state. Elsewhere, health is regarded as a commodity, and in some nations, state-of-the-art medical care is dispensed only by health maintenance organizations (HMOs), corporations whose shares are traded in the stock market. What would Hippocrates think of this?

Norm 5 (safety and informed consent) enjoins keeping the distinction between patient and guinea pig, as well as respecting the patient's (or her proxy's) right to participate in the making of life-and-death decisions. Evidently, some gravely wounded or sick persons are unable to exert this right, and so their fate rests in the hands of a paramedic or intern. When there are not enough health caregivers on the spot, as it usually happens in war and after massive accidents, the health worker is forced to practice triage, that is, to assign priorities to the injured.

Which is the fairest triaging procedure? Intuitively, the more gravely wounded should be assisted first. But in the battlefield and at the place of a disaster, when only some of the victims can be assisted, the most practical option is not to treat the dying but to dispense first aid to those with the highest survival chance. In general, the important trumps the urgent. However, triage is the subject of long discussions that we must leave to bioethics experts.

The importance of a legal or moral norm, or lack thereof, is best appreciated when breached. Let us therefore take a quick look at a few egregious cases of breach of medical ethics. Norm 5, about safety and consent, was broken not only by the notorious Nazi and Japanese concentration camp physicians; it was also breached by the American military doctors who, between 1946 and 1948, infected 1,308 Guatemalans with venereal diseases (Walter 2012). The same norm was also violated by the Russian psychiatrists who authorized the forcible confinement of political dissidents in psychiatric hospitals.

The doctors who assisted torturers of political prisoners and terrorism suspects in many Third World countries — sometimes under CIA contract — were equally guilty. But they were seldom caught and never disciplined. A rare and sensational exception was the Argentine physician who, in 1951, at the request of the political police, dispensed medical assistance to an individual who had fallen into a coma as a result of beatings and discharges from a cattle prod. The police became concerned when the "disappearance" of the student became a *cause celèbre*, and students and political opponents were mobilized. The torture victim was Ernesto Mario Bravo, a Communist chemistry student who wrote with his own blood a message on a wall of his cell. The courageous judge Conrado Sadi Massué examined the detention cell, read the message, and ordered the arrest and prosecution of the police commissioner in charge. Bravo was set free, but shortly thereafter, the Perón government pardoned the main culprit. The repentant doctor, Alberto Julián Caride, fled the country and told his *mea culpa* to the weekly *Colliers*.

A far better-known case of medical complicity with political power was that of the psychiatrist Dr. Donald Ewen Cameron and colleagues at McGill University. In the 1950s and early 1960s, they conducted some "brainwashing" (or "mind-control") experiments partially funded by the CIA. The goals were the destruction of memories and the implant of "false memories," to explain political conversion, as well as the attempt to force people to do what they don't want to do. Since consent for performing such barbaric operations was unobtainable, it was never sought. Some of these unsuspecting victims of electroshock and frequent LSD doses, like the mathematical geographer Professor William Bunge, were left incapacitated for life, others in a permanent coma.

Certain pharmaceutical companies have been conducting equally unethical experiments. They use professional human guinea pigs, who are miserably paid and not duly informed of potential risks, to find out whether their new drugs have the desired effects. Ditto the European drug companies who used unsuspecting African peasants for such purposes, as John le Carré denounced in his novel *The Constant Gardener*.

The same Norm 5 raises the minor issue of whether it is right to prescribe placebos. There are two philosophical stands on this matter. A Kantian moral philosopher will hold that the practice in question is wrong because one ought never to lie, regardless of the consequences. By contrast, utilitarians and humanists share the standard view, that lies come in two kinds: the black or harmful ones, which benefit only the liar; and the white or pious ones, which benefit someone else. Of course, we should never tell black lies. But if we wish to help people enjoy life, for example by alleviating the sufferings of terminally ill patients, there is nothing wrong with telling some inoffensive lies, as telling the naked truth may be unnecessarily cruel.

Kant's norm, to do what is right regardless of the consequences for *me*, is noble if confined to the personal sphere. But the same norm is cruel in general, for my behavior, however upright, may harm others — as is the case with the physician who refuses to inject morphine into a person dying in great pain. Moreover, non-consequentialism is also dogmatic because ethics, unlike theoretical philosophy, is the core of practical philosophy, and a practical discipline that refuses to evaluate its principles by checking the consequences of the actions suggested by those rules, is no better than a religious dogma.

How does the preceding apply to the therapeutic use of placebos, such as prescribing initially subtherapeutic doses of antidepressants? Obviously, this practice is deceitful and, if the patient discovers the truth, she will get angry and lose her trust in her doctor. What is to be done? The "official" policy is to repudiate the deliberate use of placebos, but several studies have shown that most psychiatrists use placebos with good results. This is why Foddy (2009) has argued for the "duty to deceive."

The problem in question is an instance of the conflict among values (or among norms), familiar to moral philosophers from antiquity. In the case of the therapeutic use of placebos, the pursuit of health may be incompatible with telling the truth — but not with the truth that such a practice may be beneficial. Since the first desideratum, health, trumps the patient's knowledge of the full truth of the matter, the practice in question is morally justified. Moreover, contrary to what has been maintained, that particular white lie does not go against evidence-based medicine, since randomized controlled trials have confirmed the benefits of such deceptive placebos in question (Raz *et al.* 2009).

Norm 6 (protection against sectarian demands and medical quackery) is part of the defense of modern culture from both traditional superstition and the postmodernist fad. However, in a democratic society, the most that physicians and governments can do is to warn the public that such and such precepts or practices are at best innocuous, and at worst health hazards. Unsupervised medical tourism is a case in point. About 100 Chinese firms are selling, through travel agencies, stem cell treatments for several diseases, that have neither passed randomized controlled trials nor received the stamp of approval of the Chinese sanitary authorities.

What about vaccination against contagious diseases? Should it be left to the individual's decision? Yes, according to amoralism and libertarianism. No, according to both social utilitarianism and humanism, because pathogen carriers are public enemies, as was made public in the mid-nineteenth century, when the American cook known as Typhoid Mary was forcibly isolated during three decades for infecting others with typhoid fever.

What should be done about parents who, in the name of certain religious beliefs, refuse to allow their children to receive a blood transfusion in life-threatening situations? Most judges in the advanced countries have ordered this procedure to be carried out, thereby curtailing parental power (*patria potestas*). In this case, it is admitted that parents do not own their children, and that the state has the duty to protect children against their parents' abuses or ignorance.

Finally, Norm 7 (about medical rights) has various aspects: (a) it admits that erring in good faith is human; (b) it protects physicians against unfair litigation; (c) it protects doctors against exploitation; and (d) it allows physicians to violate the norm "Do everything possible to delay death" when it would be cruel to prolong by artificial means, such as respirators, an existence that cannot possibly be enjoyed, and that has become a burden to everyone concerned.

However, these rights imply the obligation to observe the previous norms, in particular those of (a) making only prudent decisions backed by the best available medical knowledge; and (b) securing the continuation of essential medical assistance during strikes, which in turn recommends bargaining before striking, and stopping intermittently as long as negotiations continue. Physicians, like teachers, are public servants even when self-employed.

9.3 Social Medical Ethics

Social medical assistance does not concern directly individual medical practice; it is about the collective actions that aim at protecting personal well-being. These actions happen in hospitals and clinics, in biomedical research units and in pharmaceutical industries, in the street and in non-governmental organizations (NGOs), in public offices and parliaments — in short, wherever people get together to discuss or implement health care measures on a social scale.

Whistleblowing is one of the most courageous actions of this kind. Dr. Marcia Angell's (2004) denunciations of the deceptions of the drug industry, as well as of the severe flaws of the American health care system, are classics. The case of Dr. Nancy Olivieri, the Toronto hematologist disciplined in the late 1990s for blowing the whistle on a drug used to treat a blood disorder, is still remembered because it involved a conflict between scientific integrity and the interests of a pharmaceutical firm and university administrators accused of favoring the latter instead of defending academic freedom (see Shuchman 2005).

The issues of interest to social medical ethics go from triage to the rights of human guinea pigs, the distribution of acute and chronic patients among clinics and hospitals, the merger and splitting of hospitals, the production of affordable drugs, the access to public health care, and population control. These are all social issues that the socially concerned physician must face, but cannot solve by himself; they require the cooperation of physicians, managers, statesmen, and NGOs. And some of them call for public debate.

Some of the above-mentioned issues have been around since the state, particularly in ancient Rome, assumed the responsibility for public health, but have multiplied and gotten ever more complicated since the birth of the welfare state around 1900, when health care policies were submitted to public debate and the popular ballot, and when the pharmaceutical industry became as big, lucrative, and politically influential as the arms industry.

One of the hardest unresolved problems with the drug companies is how to control them in the public interest without depriving them of the pecuniary incentives that lead them to risking capital in the search for medically promising compounds. Let us glance at only a few of these issues, starting with the rights of the human guinea pigs employed in massive clinical trials. They are all destitute, marginal, and utterly powerless immigrants, who are easily persuaded to rent their bodies with no one to safeguard their health.

So far, most governments have declined to intervene in this matter, for the professional guinea pigs are marginal; they have neither family nor union, and they do not even have the right to vote. A possible solution would be to regulate the renting of the body, requiring that all clinical trials be closely supervised by the sanitary authority, hence conducted in universities or public hospitals rather than in private laboratories. But who is willing to bell this homeless and clawless cat?

Another big sociomedical problem is that only the inhabitants of the First World (about one billion people) and the upper crust of the rest (another billion) can afford to buy the most effective drugs produced by Big Pharma. The rest of humankind, some five billion humans, have no access to them, and are thus the easy prey of shamans. Besides, those big drug companies do not produce vaccines or affordable drugs to prevent or treat most of the tropical diseases, such as amebiasis, giardiasis, malaria, dengue fever, yellow fever, leprosy, and the Chagas sleeping sickness.

Thus, modern pharmacology reaches only two out of every seven human beings. But let us not blame science for this moral failure. What is to be blamed is the same regime wherein only farmers who practice subsistence agriculture welcome bumper crops; those who work for the market dislike abundance because it lowers the price of their produce. Nor is this the only one of the market "pathologies," that only the Scandinavian nations have avoided, because they have combined equality with freedom and a strong state. Physicians cannot treat those pathologies because the social body is not an organism but an artifact. But at least they can abstain from complicity.

The economic law of decreasing returns has not spared the pharmaceutical industry; although the available drugs are perfectible, increased research inputs have not produced proportional results. This is why the pharmacologists working on anticancer drugs are experiencing increasing difficulties in obtaining research grants, as Richard J. Roberts, a Nobel laureate in medicine, declared recently (Amiguet 2007). And by 2012, all but one of the big drug companies had dismantled their brain research facilities. The same holds for the production of generic drugs, those that are no longer protected by patents — free competition is good in words but not in practice.

This failure of nerve on the part of the private sector is a powerful argument for the partisans of the public ownership of drug manufacturing.

As a matter of fact, the Indian, Brazilian, and South African governments have already intervened to remedy the scarcity of key drugs, contracting their manufacturing with small laboratories. Who knows how the governments committed to the free-market ideology will handle unavoidable emergencies, such as unforeseen pandemics? Will they and their electorates finally understand that securing the supply of affordable key drugs is as serious an issue as those of security, sanitation, and education?

In conclusion, because health is, along with security and education, the most basic value, it is also the one that lends itself best to exploitation as well as to altruism. For this reason, it is desirable that both health care and the health industries be supervised by the state and NGOs: to protect the most vulnerable members of any society — children, the sick, and the elderly.

Coda

Unlike artists and basic scientists, physicians are public servants even if they are not paid by the state. This is why they are subject to legal controls on top of moral rules. In all societies, most physicians are responsible, dedicated, overworked, and sometimes self-denying as well. Most doctors do their duty not only because they are responsible persons, but also because they like what they do; their occupation is their calling. They automatically fulfill the humanist maxim, *Enjoy life and help live.*

Because of the fast pace of medical advancement and the multiplication of medical specialties, medical practice is becoming ever more demanding. Hence, complying with the medico-ethical imperative of healing or alleviating suffering is becoming increasingly difficult. Is the medic's exceptional work always duly appreciated? And is there a consensus on the nature of medicine, its place in culture, and its social role? Let us discuss these matters in the next chapter.

CHAPTER 10

SCIENCE OR TECHNOLOGY, CRAFT OR SERVICE?

10.1 The Place of Medicine in Culture

The status of medicine has been debated since Hippocrates stated that the physician is "a recognized craftsman with some knowledge of natural science." What is medicine today: science or applied science, technology, craft, or service?

To find an adequate answer to this question, let us look at what is being done in the advanced medical centers, such as university hospitals. However, before visiting any such center, it will be convenient to recall the following definitions, which involve the concept of a *discipline* as a body of rigorous and systematic knowledge rather than a mere catalog of beliefs.

Basic (or *untargeted*) *science*: Discipline cultivated by individuals who investigate knowledge problems using the scientific method, to produce new knowledge for its own sake. Examples: physics, chemistry, biology, linguistics, and history.

Applied (or *translational*) *science*: The same as basic science, except that its goal is getting truths of *possible* practical use. Examples: pharmacology and clinical psychology.

Technology (*modern*): Discipline cultivated by persons specialized in designing, improving, or repairing artificial or semi-artifical systems — such as machines, farms, persons, and formal organizations — with the help of scientific knowledge. Examples: therapeutics, normative epidemiology, bioengineering, education science, jurisprudence, and management science.

High-level craft: Manual expertise that makes intensive use of science and technology. Examples: obstetrics, surgery, and dentistry.

Service (qualified): Activity aimed at satisfying needs or wishes with the help of technological knowledge. Examples: medical practice, nursing, physiotherapy, and social work.

A guided tour of a large advanced medical center or medical school will show that, whereas some of its members do basic science, others do applied science, and still others technology, craft, or service. A few medical centers also include scholars working in some of the medical humanities and biosocial sciences and technologies, in particular bioethics, medical anthropology, sociology, economics and history, and forensic medicine.

Obviously, then, medicine is not a unidiscipline but a *multidiscipline*; it is a variegated system of fields of knowledge and practices centered in health care as both a branch of knowledge and a practice. In fact, in any large advanced medical center, one will meet persons working in any of these fields:

- *basic biomedical sciences*: biophysics, biochemistry, molecular biology, genetics, cytology, anatomy, physiology, endocrinology, immunology, and neuroscience;
- *applied (or translational) biomedical sciences*: bacteriology, virology, parasitology, pharmacology, toxicology, and descriptive epidemiology;
- *biomedical technologies*: design of new therapies, medicaments, prostheses, and surgical procedures;
- *medical crafts:* anesthesia, obstetrics, nursing, and physiotherapy;
- *sociomedical technologies*: normative (prescriptive) epidemiology, social medicine, and hospital administration; and
- *medical humanities*: medical ethics, medical anthropology and sociology, history and philosophy of medicine, and forensic medicine.

Figure 10.1 exhibits the place of medicine in the system of rigorous knowledge and qualified skills.

All the categories of medical knowledge and skills, except for that of applied science, are fairly well understood. In particular, it is well known that, whereas basic scientists try to understand the world, technologists seek

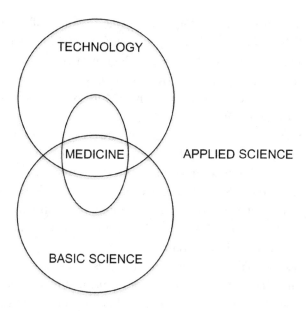

Fig. 10.1. Medicine is in the intersection of basic science and technology.

to transform it. By contrast, the concept of applied (or translational) science has been neglected and even misunderstood to the point that it is often confused with that of technology. To check whether pharmacology fits the definition of applied science proposed above, let us look at what pharmacologists do.

Clearly, there are two main kinds of pharmacological work: seeking to *understand* the composition and mechanism of action of drugs on organisms, and *designing* new drugs, or new uses for known drugs. While the workers of both types are expected to proceed scientifically, the drug designers are technologists, just like the creative engineers and designers of social policies. By contrast, the former, even if they do not seek practical results, they do not engage in basic or disinterested research, for they confine their interest to the possible pharmacodynamic action of chemicals on the health of animals, especially humans and plants; they look for truths of *possible* medical, industrial, or agricultural interest.

Thus, pharmacology is part technology and part applied science. Without disease, there would be no medicine; and without medicine, there would be no pharmacology, while there would still be chemistry, biology, and biochemistry — as any objective report on Shangri-La will attest. Admittedly, however, the epistemological categories in question are somewhat fuzzy because there are overlaps among them, which is a source of confusion and inconclusive argument. (More on the various types of knowledge in Bunge 1983.)

The distinctions we have drawn above are psychologically and philosophically interesting but of little practical import, for the quality of the product trumps the motivation of the production process. As the Dean of the Harvard Medical School recently put it, "All research should be assessed by one criterion: the novelty, importance, and impact of the insights generated" (Flier 2013). Let us then peep into the conditions favorable to excellence in research.

A common yet false belief is that all that is needed to conduct high-level research is state-of-the-art laboratories manned by competent scientists. This does hold for "Big Science," like the one that gave us the sequencing of the human DNA. But "Small Science," the one that individuals and small teams conduct, needs mainly brain power. Yet, in either case, instruments big or small would be useless in hands guided by an uneducated and unoriginal brain. For this reason, anyone planning to set up a scientific center should begin by recruiting good brains instead of ordering instruments by the catalog; the investigators will tell the organizer what they need. For the same reason, in every productive laboratory, lab technicians help researchers handle the experimental equipment.

A technician may have manual skills that the original investigator lacks, even if he designed the piece of apparatus handled by the former. What holds for the laboratory also holds, *mutatis mutandis*, for the hospital. For instance, it is well known that nurses are more skillful than doctors at changing bandages, giving injections, or cheering up the sick and easing their death.

What is less well known is that nurses, in addition to being skillful and compassionate craftspersons, are the ones who make the hospital tick as a unit around the patients. As Lewis Thomas (1983: 67) put it, "The institution [hospital] is held together, *glued* together, enabled to function as an organism, by the nurses and by nobody else." The reason is that they are the ones who care for patients from start to finish as surrogate mothers, ferry them through the hospital's labyrinth, and keep their files.

Doctors know *what* must be done to patients, but only nurses know *how* to do it competently. Incidentally, it was philosophers, notably Bertrand Russell, who first noted and studied the differences between *know-what* and *know-how*, or knowledge by description (or explicit and from books) and knowledge by acquaintance (or tacit and from experience), respectively. But only developmental psychologists are equipped to learn how; with experience, know-what may gradually become know-how; as in the case of surgeons.

Medical education, the focus of the influential Flexner Report (1910) and a regular feature in the *Journal of the American Medical Association*, has recently become a philosophical minefield. In particular, many American medical schools have adopted the *Dreyfus model* of acquisition of medical skills, without examining its philosophical pedigree. That "model," or rather doctrine, postulates that medicine is only a skill, so that learning medicine does not differ from learning skills like aircraft piloting (Dreyfus & Dreyfus 1980). This doctrine is alien to education science, and it does not invoke any empirical studies on the ways that medicine was taught since the birth of modern medical schools at around 1800.

Indeed, the Dreyfus model only relies on the alleged authority of Husserl's phenomenology and Heidegger's existentialism (Peña 2010). Both schools exalt intuition or gut feeling, denigrate reason, and oppose science, and Heidegger held that all mental work is handwork. Neither Husserl nor Heidegger offered any evidence for their opaque theses, and neither of them ever showed any interest in medicine.

In his masterpiece *Madame Bovary*, Gustave Flaubert criticized *avant la lettre* the opinion that medicine is only a manual skill, when he invented the rural medic Charles Bovary. This ignorant and dull man wished to gain a reputation as a great surgeon by attempting to correct an inborn deformity without having the requisite anatomical knowledge, and only succeeded in worsening it.

A far more important but harmless confusion between knowledge and skill was the one involved in the birth of nursing schools that offer postgraduate programs and diplomas, and whose professors qualify for research grants. There are even manuals for crafting nursing theories — whatever these may be. The very idea that it is possible to teach how to construct theories, particularly in a field that is not known for its theoretical wealth, is proof of the inventiveness of adventurers.

The idea of an *ars inveniendi* has been around since about 1600, and it is still a mirage pursued by some computer scientists — though of course there are no programs for the invention of computer programs or of anything else. The reason for such inability to invent should be obvious: machines lack spontaneity and creativity, and they work only when guided step by step, either by hand or by program. Back to nursing education.

No doubt, it was high time to admit the importance and nobility of the nursing profession. But does this craft really benefit from separating its apprenticeship from that of medicine and attempting to pass it off as a science? And does health care benefit from subverting a social hierarchy based on a knowledge hierarchy? In all the other fields, craftsmen are appreciated without academic pomp. For example, we all respect good parents, cabinet-makers, plumbers, electricians, lab technicians, pilots, and actors although they do not pursue academic degrees. Doctorates in parenthood? In plumbing?

Craftsmen learn mainly on the job rather than from books or in research labs. And lab technicians and nurses are maximally efficient when working under the supervision of experienced doctors or imaginative investigators with a solid and broad background, as well as being reasonably up to date with the specialized literature. The attempt to upgrade skill to knowledge may reach the ridiculous extreme of conferring doctorates in different types of welding, as happened in the former Soviet Union (Graham 1981).

Let us now tackle another frequent confusion. The expression *medical technology* names the set of medical appliances. This usage is incorrect, because the technologies are knowledge fields, not artifacts. For example, a bioengineer invents or improves artifacts used in the biosciences, such as prostheses and instruments to measure biological parameters. Some of these artifacts are used to investigate, and others to treat patients.

The design of medical instruments and therapies requires not only ingenuity but also a lot of basic knowledge. It suffices to think of two groups of artifacts: brain-imaging devices and electronic prostheses. The design of the computerized scanner (CT) involved the solution of a complex inverse problem: that of transforming a stack of two-dimensional images ("slices") into a three-dimensional one. And the design of the magnetic resonance imaging (MRI) apparatus required some nuclear physics in addition to some neurophysiology.

The latest neuroprosthesis allows a tetraplegic to make skillful and coordinated reach-and-grasp movements by just willing to do so; the trick is done by two complex electrodes implanted in the motor cortex and connected to an artificial arm (Collinger *et al.* 2013). The dualist's claim that this only proves the power of mind on matter crumbles the moment the electrodes are inactivated, for they bridge two cortical regions: the one that does the willing and the one that controls movement. The process is thoroughly material.

These artifacts should have attracted the attention of philosophers of mind, because their very design presupposes the materialist hypothesis that the mental processes are neural. Regrettably, the vast majority of philosophers of mind have ignored the philosophical basis of neuroengineering. They have even ignored the birth of this new discipline, which resulted from the merger of three different fields: neuroscience, medicine, and engineering (see, e.g., DiLorenzo & Bronzino 2008).

10.2 Quality and Accessibility

The prodigious conceptual and practical wealth of contemporary medicine accounts for the great variety of people it attracts, from curious researchers to health missionaries to businesspeople. Whatever their initial motivation, from curiosity to pecuniary gain, they will do good if they help control disease or alleviate suffering. However, the Medicine–Money–Politics triad is unstable, so we should keep an eye on it to prevent medicine from being smothered by either of its partners-rivals. Similar conflicts occur, of course, in all of the so-called liberal professions, particularly in the law, and sometimes they call for the intervention of ethical boards.

In these matters, the moral and practical solution will be a compromise between private and public interests. The ideal is to earn a decent living by serving the community. Totally or partially socialized medicine, as practiced in the UK, Canada, and the Scandinavian nations, has been welcomed by most doctors as well as by the electorates. (Incidentally, the British doctors were from the start the most eloquent defenders of socialized medicine, whereas the American Medical Association has always opposed it.) Under this regime, the state pays for all medical expenses. As a result, no one is left without health care, physicians do not overcharge, unnecessary surgery is avoided, paper work and the cost to the taxpayer are minimal — and there is never talk of money between doctor and patient.

All the responsible physicians have sought to dispense *the best medical assistance to the greatest number*. This is a variation on the utilitarian desideratum formulated in the mid-eighteenth century by Claude Helvétius, the great materialist philosopher, and adopted by Jeremy Bentham, the influential legal and political philosopher. It is also the philosophical basis of socialized medicine.

Regrettably, the two desiderata, "best assistance" and "greatest number," are mutually incompatible, because the pie to be distributed, in our case health care, is finite. In fact, call P the size of the health budget, and divide it into n equal parts, each of them with area m, representative of the medical cost per capita. (Think of the equitable division of a pizza.) Since $P = nm$, it is impossible to maximize both m and n at once. True, both factors increase every time the health budget increases. But P cannot increase indefinitely, hence health care has got to be rationed, as well as charged to whoever may pay for it. However, help is on its way.

Actually, the problem is far less serious than suggested above, because medical costs vary with individuals; roughly half of the population only requires preventive medicine, whereas about two-thirds of all health spending is consumed by the 10% made up of the chronically ill and the terminally ill. In other words, the assumption that there is a single health care cost m for everyone is false; in a well-organized society, the healthy pay for the sick. Insurance of any kind is parallel — the lucky and careful pay for the unlucky and careless.

Nowadays, in many advanced nations, the health budget is held constant or has started to decrease, because it has competitors with more clout, such as "defense" and the service of the fiscal debt. And the populations of the underdeveloped nations keep increasing, so that there are never enough health care facilities, schools, or other public resources.

In short, nearly everywhere, there is an unresolved conflict between the quality and the quantity of public health care. Good physicians refuse to make concessions with regard to quality, and responsible hospital managers are forced to ration resources. How can this conflict be resolved? The orthodox economists — those who cling to an old theory that has never explained, much less predicted, any economic crisis — propose commodifying health care and abolishing all the sanitary services. They do not care that nobody profits from the bad health of the majority; they have never heard of contagious diseases or of epidemics, or even of the lower productivity and morale of sick workers. The orthodox economists constitute a clear example of the dangers of sectoral outlooks and the disregard for morals.

Another sectoral approach to the rising costs of health care is the claim of the leaders of EBM (evidence-based medicine) that to check such costs it would suffice to employ only therapies that have passed rigorous clinical trials (Sackett *et al.* 1996). True but insufficient: the issue of the conflict between the quality of health care and its accessibility is neither strictly medical nor purely one of management: that is a bulky social problem, in particular a political one. Let us see why.

The issue in question is social and therefore multifaceted; it lies at the intersection of several fields, from medicine to politics, and therefore it calls for a systemic approach instead of a sectoral one. I submit that the solution is a whole package of social policies, including (a) planned parenthood; (b) a substantial rise in the human development index and a significant drop in the income inequality index; (c) reinforcement of preventive medicine; (d) a far more effective dietetic and hygienic education; (e) easier access to healthy housing in healthy environments; (f) stronger environmental protection; (g) price control of pharmaceutical drugs; (h) reinforcement of the NGOs (non-governmental organizations) working on health problems; and (i) far more intensive political participation of the citizenry, so that it may force statesmen and politicians to adopt and respect the above-listed measures.

The proposed reforms amount to a radical social change, though not as radical as the failed revolutions and counter-revolutions of the past century. Indeed, every one of the reforms we propose has been enacted in some of the advanced nations; what is new in our proposal is that it joins all the partial social reforms. If anyone were to object to it, one might retort with this question: what should we prefer, to own more or to feel better, to stand taller in the world or to coexist peacefully?

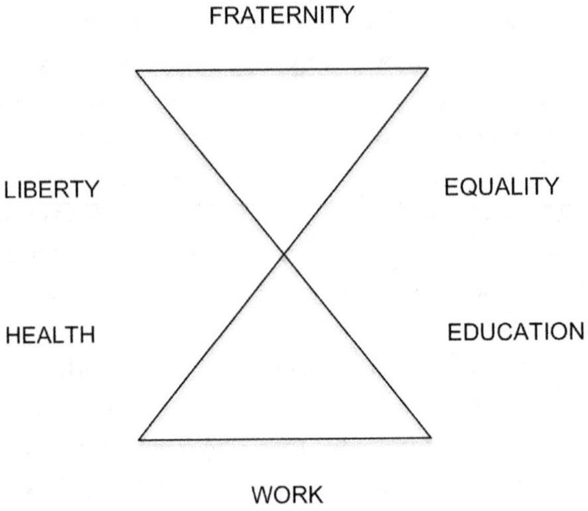

FRATERNITY

LIBERTY   EQUALITY

HEALTH   EDUCATION

WORK

Fig. 10.2. The political triad (equality–liberty–fraternity) rests on the biosocial one (work–health–education).

The problem at hand belongs in political philosophy and it is studied in academic institutions, but the place to work on it and fight for it is in the political arena. However, politics as usual is insufficient for debating or settling any social problems, because those politics are mostly confined to political values. Not even the admirable slogan of the French revolutionaries of 1789 — *Liberté, égalité, fraternité* — is enough. It is insufficient because it overlooks the fact that the people expected to enact it must be educated and enjoy good health on top of having jobs — *primum vivere* and all that. These three factors are interdependent and they constitute the tripod on which the political triad must rest. (See Figure 10.2.)

10.3 Diagnosis and Prognosis of Medicine

The advances of medicine have been sensational since about 1800. But this discipline has not reached perfection, nor is there any reason that the practice of medicine will ever become as automatized as banking operations. Medical problems can never become routine problems, because there are no two identical persons; because different people react differently to any given treatment; and because medical knowledge, though huge, is not always deep, and will always be imperfect. It suffices to recall the new diseases spread by war, tourism, and migrations; the problems of dosing and of the interactions among medications; or the issue of the rising cost of health care.

The champions of EBM seem to believe that they started a new medical era characterized by far more rigorous assays, and by data-driven rather than by hypotheses-driven research. This tendency is neither new nor healthy, because it has only strengthened the empiricist tendency to accumulate undigested data and mistrust all theory. What but new intriguing hypotheses can motivate and guide the search for data of a new kind? For instance, why study the brain unless one suspects that it does something important? Or why keep studying it despite the current deceleration of psychoneuropharmacology, unless one suspects that new hypotheses are conceivable and badly needed?

As stressed in the first two chapters, all medicines, in contradistinction to shamanic lore, have been based on data, though not always true or important data. This virtue can be exaggerated to the point of becoming swamped by data that make no sense because of the lack of theories. A mature science, like physics or chemistry, has two foci: a database and a body of theories capable of explaining those data and guiding further original research.

The nucleus of a scientific theory is a set of *law statements*, that is, precise and well-confirmed propositions about objective regularities or patterns, such as the course of a disease or the evolution of an epidemic. Some scientific laws are *universal*; they hold for entire genera of things. Others, the so-called *constitutive* laws, hold only for stuff of special kinds. Genetics and evolutionary biology, just like physics and chemistry, contain laws of both kinds. By contrast, medicine can boast of very few laws of either kind. The laws about the flow of blood are often cited as examples of medical laws, but actually they belong in physiology rather than in medicine, because they do not concern any pathologies. A medical law proper will be about the onset or the course of a disease.

Laws are not found by accumulating empirical data, but by thinking hard and deeply about the salient features of facts of some kind, which is why neither computation experts nor their machines can find any. For example, it was not a detailed medical study of cretins that led to understanding the cause and cure of cretinism. This terrible disorder was explained by a research project triggered by a typically scientific question: what are the specific functions of the thyroid glands? Research suggested that cretinism is caused by thyroid insufficiency, which can be corrected with a thyroid extract. This finding was an unexpected practical bonus of disinterested endocrinological research.

Likewise, dwarfism and gigantism were not explained by examining dwarves and giants. These serious congenital anomalies were understood only by studying the pituitary gland (or hypophysis), which synthesizes the growth hormone. And why was this gland singled out? Because it was known that this is a multitask organ; it secretes hormones of nine different kinds, every one of which helps control a key function in all vertebrates, from growth and metabolism to body temperature and blood pressure. So, it was only natural to conjecture that the pituitary gland is involved in dwarfism and gigantism.

In short, an intriguing hypothesis, true or false, may be fruitful in suggesting the search for (actually production of) important data, some of which may support or undermine the hypothesis, which is why they deserve being promoted from neutral *data* to *evidence*. For example, the datum that this fellow, normally self-controlled and peaceful, has lately been unusually aggressive, points to hyperthyroidism as the prime suspect. A lab analysis will put this hypothesis to the test, and move the physician to either mess with the patient's thyroid or drop the case. As long as the lab results are not in, the hypothesis in question will be more or less plausible in light of the extant knowledge, but it is not yet either true or false. An untestable hypothesis will never acquire a truth value. And if testable, the body of relevant evidence (theoretical as well as empirical) will grow to the point where the hypothesis can be said to be true or false — until further notice.

(The preceding statements on truth and falsity being "acquired characteristics" of some propositions are at variance with the standard or Platonic view of the matter, that all propositions are true or false from conception. But the history of science does not corroborate this view, which may be called "alethic nativism," for history shows that many hypotheses are true only to a first approximation, and that further research may either discard them or suggest alternative hypotheses that are assigned a greater or lesser truth value.)

So far, we have dealt only with isolated hypotheses. Theories, or hypothetico-deductive systems, are far stronger than isolated hypotheses, because every constituent of a theory is supported or weakened by every other component. Regrettably, as remarked above, medicine is very poor in theories — most of its hypotheses are isolated. And yet, it stands to reason that diseases, being processes involving many interrelated and changing properties, would be best represented by conceptual networks such as systems of equations.

There are a few successful mathematical models of particular diseases, such as the chaos-theoretic model of cardiac arrhythmia proposed by Mackey and Glass (1988), and the adverse hematopoietic effects of chemotherapy (Brooks *et al.* 2012). However, nearly all the mathematical models of diseases are but mathematizations of empirical curves, so that they throw no light on the mechanisms of action, and thus, they have no explanatory power. Medicine is thus at a pre-Newtonian level. Should the medical counterpart of Newton emerge, would he/she be recognized as such? This is uncertain, because of the chasm between medical schools and mathematics departments, as a result of which the papers in mathematical medicine appear in biology journals rather than in medical ones. Another powerful contributing cause is the prevalent data-and-computer cult.

The ideal of some bioinformatics experts is to digitalize all the extant medical knowledge, and put it on the Internet, thus, that everyone may diagnose and medicate themselves, hence vacating hospital beds and saving on health care costs. These dreamers forget that the most important biomarkers are inaccessible to lay people, so that even the most complete medical expert system would be of little use to individuals who, at best, can describe what they feel, seldom what really ails them, and much less what they need.

May we expect that medicine will keep advancing at the speed it attained in the last century? This is not sure, because medicine is propelled by biomedical research, and researchers need support as well as curious and disciplined brains. But support for basic research has been decreasing in recent years, because science has lost the popularity it used to enjoy in the mid-twentieth century, when even politicians understood that science is the main fountain of modern culture, when the pharmaceutical industry was still investing heavily in research, and when postmodernism was just starting its crusade against rationality.

There are signs that the glittering party of science and science-intensive technology, which tovarich Sputnik unwittingly launched half a century ago, may soon be over. Indeed, science budgets are suffering more and more cuts, and bright minds, in increasing numbers, are devoting more time to playing with electronic gadgets than to wondering about the world or tinkering in the garage — as indicated by the decline of enrollments in science and engineering programs. Another troubling indicator is that the vast majority of new drugs developed in the course of the last decade are tweakings to existing drugs, and what the pharmaceutical industry invests in looking for new molecules has dropped to about 1.3% of their revenues, which amounts to a ratio of basic research to marketing of 1:19 (Light & Lexchin 2012).

For any science to flourish, it must be strongly supported by society, and it must attract some of the brightest young brains in each generation. Besides, to imagine ambitious and promising research projects, scientific workers must adopt, at least tacitly, a world vision favorable to the search for truth: see Figure 10.3.

Let us put to the test the pentagon hypothesis, imagining what would happen if any of its sides were erased.

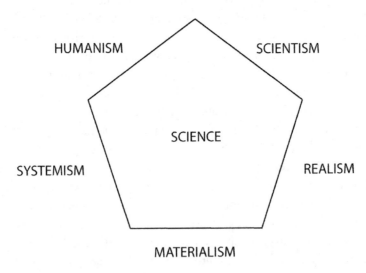

Fig. 10.3. The philosophical matrix of scientific progress (from Bunge 2012a: 28).

Without materialism, both diseases and therapies would be taken to be purely spiritual.

Without systemism, every disease would be attributed to an independent module.

Without realism, diseases would be viewed as either imaginary or as social flaws.

Without scientism, either nihilism or dogmatism would prevail, and all the achievements of biomedical research of the last 500 years would be consigned to oblivion.

Without humanism, all medical practice would be mercenary, and there would be no public health care.

All five scenarios can be found somewhere nowadays. Indeed, (a) spiritualist medicines are still being practiced by shamans and cult followers; (b) the sectoral approach is still being adopted to tackle systemic problems like those of hypertension, diabetes, and public health; (c) social constructivism, which holds diseases to be either inventions of the medical profession or iatrogenic (effects of medical practices), is still going strong; (d) the "complementary and alternative medicines" enjoy more prestige and more customers than a century ago; and (e) doctors, in increasing numbers, are employees of "health maintenance organizations" whose shares are traded in stock markets, and torturers always find medics to assist them.

I submit that the vast majority of physicians and biomedical researchers operate inside the pentagon, and medicine is still so prestigious that it is reasonable to expect new spectacular medical advances. But it would be foolish to attempt to prophesy them. All that can be done is to list some of the advances that are not only desirable but also possible in view of present knowledge. Here are a few: (a) strengthening the convergence of the various biomedical sciences along with their multiplication; (b) continuing to invent artificial parts, such as blood, skin, hearts, and neuroprostheses; (c) encouraging the development of drugs to treat diseases endemic to underdeveloped nations; (d) fostering the invention of realistic medical theories (hypothetico-deductive systems of statements); and (e) filling the gap between medicine for the rich and medicine for the poor, as pointed out by the Persian polymath Razi, working in Baghdad in the ninth century of our era.

Where is the philosophical pentagon being studied? Do not look for it in the faculties of humanities, for these have always preferred erudition to original research, and dead authors to live problems. And nowadays, the most widely read authors in the humanities — notably Hegel, Nietzsche, Bergson, Dilthey, Husserl, Heidegger, Wittgenstein, and Foucault — were hostile or indifferent to science and technology. Most of the pro-science philosophers, from Descartes to Russell, have thrived outside academia. For example, the influential *philosophes* of the French Enlightenment met at the *salons* of d'Holbach, Helvétius, or Quesnay, not at the Sorbonne.

The advantage of academic marginality is freedom to think and discuss heterodoxies. But the disadvantage of such marginality is that the knowledge of amateurs tends to be spotty because they read what they want, not what they need. However, collaboration in the laboratory and discussion in the seminar are always possible, and they can correct such deficiencies. In particular, biomedical researchers can help invent medical theories if they collaborate with mathematicians, and they can broaden their horizons if they collaborate with pro-science philosophers.

Coda

The idea that there is such a thing as medical philosophy is likely to shock philosophers and medics alike. Therefore, it should be discussed in historical perspective. The traditional views about the philosophy–science connection are that (a) they are two well-demarcated and mutually independent domains and (b) philosophy should orient or even oversee scientific endeavors. I trust that this book has confuted both views, in showing that medicine and its practice are chock-full of philosophical assumptions; that philosophers have much to learn from science and technology; and that they can help medics clear up confusions, ask intriguing questions that have escaped medical specialists, and encourage medics to invest more time in theory-building, as well as in debunking pseudo-medicines and in protecting themselves against pseudophilosophies and pseudosociologies.

The idea that both medical research and practice thrive only when conducted inside the philosophical pentagon depicted in Figure 10.3 is extravagant at first sight. We will argue now that the very existence of

scientific medicine is jeopardized as soon as any of the sides of this pentagon is erased.

1) The physicians who disbelieve the independent existence of their
patients won't treat or charge them. Thus, anti-realism is an obstacle
to medical practice and public health.

2) Some postmodern authors have denied that diseases are real. In particular, the anti-psychiatry movement was based on the opinion that
what pass for mental disorders are only social dysfunctions (see
Shorter 1997). But of course, the brain can get sick, just like any
other organ, whereas society cannot, except metaphorically. It is also
obvious that, if all mental disorders were imaginary, anyone could
feel and behave sanely or insanely at will.

3) The radical skeptics, like Sextus Empiricus in antiquity and Francisco
Sánches in the Renaissance, denied that anything might be known.
David Hume and Immanuel Kant, as well as their positivist followers,
held that things can only be known in their perceptible manifestations.
So, had they written about medicine, they would have claimed that
only the symptoms of diseases are knowable and would have rejected
the very idea of an imperceptible mechanism. Karl Popper, the most
popular of contemporary skeptics, maintained that all knowledge is con-
jectural: that even the existence of the Sun is only hypothetical — which
of course leads to inaction. This is not how scientists think: they do not
question everything at once because, to think up a research project and
write a research grant, one must assume that the things to be studied exist
or may exist; nor do they doubt the existence of their laboratory and its
surroundings. The researcher also assumes that the bulk of his scientific
knowledge, or at least the part of it which that he uses to formulate his
research questions, is correct at least to a first approximation. The reason for this is purely logical: every problem belongs to some body of
knowledge, outside which it does not even make sense. For example, a
doctor will not investigate the possibility that a broken bone heals
because of a placebo effect, because he knows that the brain — the
source of the placebo effect — does not control bone repair.

4) If we denied that diseases have objective indicators, we could never
know with certainty that they occur, and consequently would not

seek to treat them as real biological processes deserving anything more than the relief of symptoms.

5) Consistent social constructivist-relativists, if there are any, do not consult physicians, because they deny that these may know any objective truths about diseases and therapies. But of course, the constructivists themselves tacitly admit that truths of this kind may be known when they claim that, truly, there are no truths.

So far, our remarks have concerned ontology and epistemology, the two foci of theoretical philosophy. The following remarks will also touch on praxiology (action theory).

6) The maxim *All diseases are treatable* belongs to the medical profession of faith. It is confirmed every time an effective therapy is found, and challenged every time no such course of action is found. But the principle is irrefutable, because it enables us to shift the goal indefinitely. (As Kant would have said, it is not a constitutive principle but a regulative one.)

7) The principle that diseases should be treated with material means, rather than by appealing to spiritual powers, is part of the philosophical materialism inherent in medicine from Hippocrates on. The principle is at variance with the spiritualism that characterizes shamanism, Christian Science, homeopathy, and other "alternative medicines." Contemporary physicians do not perform spiritual rituals, and the X-ray machines in Turkish hospitals are handled and repaired as machines working on purely physical principles, even if they are decorated with amulets to avert the "evil eye." However, psychiatrists may combine pills with talking therapies, because they trust that reasonable advice about habits and social relations helps when it strikes receptive brains. But they know that patients will follow their advice only if they like it.

8) Because knowledge is fallible, all therapies are perfectible or even discardable in light of new research findings. And every therapy must pass rigorous clinical trials before being adopted, because effectiveness relies on truth, not faith. This methodological norm is the basis of the Hippocratic Oath, which enjoins the physician to offer help and avoid harm.

9) The distinction between deep and superficial therapies corresponds to the difference between mechanisms of action and symptoms. It also matches the key distinction, drawn by Galileo and adopted by Descartes and Locke, between *primary properties* (such as wavelength and temperature) and *secondary properties* (such as color and thermal sensation). For example, colors are not in the external world, but emerge in the normal brain, usually in reaction to luminous stimuli. Physics cannot explain colors, but cognitive neuroscience can. Hence, the occurrence of secondary properties or *qualia* refutes physicalism, but not systemic and emergent materialism.

10) Prescientific healers knew a few things, but it was only recently that their hits have been accounted for in a scientific manner. For instance, vaccination is one of the few accomplishments of traditional Indian, Chinese, and Ottoman medicines. But only modern immunology explained how it works, namely by "challenging" the immune system to synthetize the antibodies that will successfully "fight" the inoculated viruses.

To sum up, medicine is chock-full of philosophy. Yet, physicians and philosophers have always ignored each other. This mutual ignorance has spared medicine contagion with the anti-science philosophers. But adherence to shallow philosophy has also involved medicine's chronic philosophical ailment, namely radical empiricism. This philosophy is hostile to theorizing, particularly about imperceptible entities and processes — the very fountains of disease and targets of medical drugs.

Rx: Just as an anti-science philosophy is bound to obstruct the advancement of medicine, a rational, realist, materialist, systemic, and humanistic one is likely to help avoiding serious blunders, as well as designing fruitful biomedical research projects and effective public health policies. It has been said that William Osler, the great clinician and educator, adopted this motto: *Ne timeas recte philosophando* — fear not, as long as you philosophize rightly.

REFERENCES

Agrest, Alberto. 2011. *En busca de la sensatez en medicina*. Buenos Aires: Zorzal.

American Psychiatric Association. 2013. *Diagnostic and Statistical Manual of Mental Disorders*, 5th ed. Washington, DC: American Psychiatric Association.

Amiguet, Lluís. 2007. Interview with Richard J. Roberts. *La Vanguardia* (Barcelona), 31 July 2007.

Anderson, Philip Warren. 1972. More is different. *Science* 172: 393–396.

Andreoli, Thomas E. *et al.* 2010. *Cecil Essentials of Medicine*. Philadelphia: Saunders Elsevier.

Angell, Marcia. 2004. *The Truth About the Drug Companies: How They Deceive Us and What to Do About It*. New York: Random House.

Ayer, A[lfred] J[ules], ed. 1959. *Logical Positivism*. Glencoe: Free Press.

Babini, José. 1950. *Historia de la medicina*. Buenos Aires: Gedisa.

Bacon, Francis. 1905. *Philosophical Works*. London: George Routledge.

Balibar, Étienne & John Rajchman, eds. 2011. *French Philosophy Since 1945*. New York & London: The New Press.

Bausell, R. Barker. 2007. *Snake Oil Science: The Truth About Complementary and Alternative Medicine*. New York: Oxford University Press.

Benedetti, Fabrizio. 2009. *Placebo Effects: Understanding the Mechanisms in Health and Disease*. New York: Oxford University Press.

Berkeley, George. 1710. *Treatise Concerning the Principles of Human Knowledge*. In A. Campbell Fraser, ed. *Works*, Vol. 1. Oxford: Clarendon Press, 1901.

Bernard, Claude. 1865. *Introduction à l'étude de la médecine expérimentale*. Paris: Flammarion, 1952.

Berry, Donald A. & Dalene Stangl, eds. 1996. *Bayesian Biostatistics*. New York: Marcel Dekker.

Bertalanffy, Ludwig von. 1950. An outline of general systems theory. *British Journal for the Philosophy of Science* 1: 139–164.

Blackburn, Elizabeth H. & Elissa S. Epel. 2012. Too toxic to ignore. *Nature* 490: 169–171.

Bleyer, Archie & H. Gilbert Welch. 2012. Effect of three decades of screening mammography on breast-cancer incidence. *New England Journal of Medicine* doi:10.1056/NEJMoa-1206809

Bliss, Michael. 1984. *The Discovery of Insulin*. Chicago: University of Chicago Press.

———. 1999. *William Osler: A Life in Medicine*. Toronto: University of Toronto Press.

———. 2011. *The Making of Modern Medicine*. Toronto: University of Toronto Press.

Blitz, David. 1992. *Emergent Evolution and the Levels of Reality*. Dordrecht & Boston: Kluwer.

Block, Ned, Owen Flanagan, & Güven Gülzedere, eds. 2002. *The Nature of Consciousness: Philosophical Debates*. Cambridge: MIT Press.

Blom, Philipp. 2010. *A Wicked Company: The Forgotten Radicalism of the European Enlightenment*. New York: Basic Books.

Bluhm, Robyn & Kristin Borgerson. 2011. Evidence-based medicine. In F. Gifford, ed. *Handbook of Philosophy of Science*, Vol. 16: *Philosophy of Medicine*, pp. 203–238. Amsterdam: Elsevier.

Boorse, Christopher. 2011. Concepts of health and disease. In F. Gifford, ed. *Handbook of Philosophy of Science*, Vol. 16: *Philosophy of Medicine*, pp. 13–64. Amsterdam: Elsevier.

Boyd, Robert & Peter J. Richerson. 1985. *Culture and the Evolutionary Process*. Chicago: University of Chicago Press.

Bradford Hill, Austin. 1937. *A Short Textbook of Medical Statistics*. 11th ed. London: Edward Arnold, 1984.

———. 1965. The environment and disease: Association or causation? *Proceedings of the Royal Society of Medicine* 58: 295–300.

Brooks, Grace, Gabriel Provencher, Jinzhi Lei, & Michael C. Mackey. 2012. Neutrophil dynamics after chemotherapy and GM-CSF: The role of pharmacokinetics in shaping the response. *Journal of Theoretical Biology* 315: 97–109.

Bunge, Mario. 1951. What is chance? *Science and Society* 15: 209–231.

———. 1959a. *Causality in Modern Science*. Repr., New York: Dover, 1979a.

———. 1959b. *Metascientific Queries*. Springfield: Charles C. Thomas.

———. 1962. *Intuition and Science*. Englewood Cliffs: Prentice Hall.

———. 1967. *Scientific Research*. 2 vols. Rev. ed., *Philosophy of Science*. New Brunswick: Transaction, 1998.

———. 1968. The maturation of science. In I. Lakatos & A. Musgrave, eds., *Problems in the Philosophy of Science*, pp. 120–137, 138–147. Amsterdam: North Holland.

———. 1969. The metaphysics, epistemology and methodology of levels. In L.L. Whyte, A.G. Wilson, & D. Wilson, eds. *Hierarchical Levels*, pp. 17–28. New York: American Elsevier.

———. 1973. *Method, Model and Matter*. Dordrecht: Reidel.

———. 1974a. *Treatise on Basic Philosophy: Semantics* 1. Dordrecht: Reidel.

———. 1974b. *Treatise on Basic Philosophy: Semantics* 2. Dordrecht: Reidel.

———. 1977a. Levels and reduction. *American Journal of Physiology: Regulatory, Integrative and Comparative Physiology* 2: 75–82.

———. 1977b. Emergence and the mind. *Neuroscience* 2: 501–509.

———. 1977c. *Treatise on Basic Philosophy*, Vol. 3: *The Furniture of the World*. Dordrecht: Reidel.

———. 1979. *Treatise on Basic Philosophy*, Vol. 4: *A World of Systems*. Dordrecht: Reidel.

———. 1980. *The Mind–Body Problem*. Oxford: Pergamon.

———. 1983. *Treatise on Basic Philosophy*, Vol. 6: *Understanding the World*. Dordrecht: Reidel.

———. 1989.*Treatise on Basic Philosophy*, Vol. 8: *Ethics: The Good and the Right*. Dordrecht & Boston: Reidel.

———. 1996a. *Finding Philosophy in Social Science*. New Haven: Yale University Press.

———. 1996b. In praise of intolerance to charlatanism in academia. *Annals of the New York Academy of Sciences* 775: 96–116.

———. 1998a. *Philosophy of Science*. 2 vols. New Brunswick: Transaction. Rev. ed. of *Scientific Research*, 2 vols. (Springer, 1967.)

———. 1998b. *Social Science under Discussion*. Toronto: University of Toronto Press.

———. 1999. *The Sociology–Philosophy Connection*. New Brunswick: Transaction.

———. 2000. Physicians ignore philosophy at their risk — and ours. *Facta Philosophica* 2: 149–160.

———. 2003a. *Emergence and Convergence*. Toronto: University of Toronto Press.

———. 2003b. *Philosophical Dictionary*. Enlarged ed. Amherst: Prometheus Books.

———. 2004. How does it work? The search for explanatory mechanisms. *Philosophy of the Social Sciences* 34: 182–210.

———. 2006. *Chasing Reality: Strife Over Realism*. Toronto: University of Toronto Press.

———. 2008. Bayesianism: Science or pseudoscience? *International Review of Victimology* 15: 169–182.

——. 2009. *Political Philosophy: Fact, Fiction, and Vision*. New Brunswick: Transaction.

——. 2010. *Matter and Mind*, Vol. 287: *Boston Studies in the Philosophy of Science*. Dordrecht, Heidelberg, London, & New York: Springer.

——. 2012a. *Evaluating Philosophies*, Vol. 295: *Boston Studies in the Philosophy of Science*. Dordrecht, Heidelberg, London, & New York: Springer.

——. 2012b. Wealth and well-being, economic growth, and integral development. *International Journal of Health Services* 42: 65–76.

Bunge, Mario & Rubén Ardila. 1987. *Philosophy of Psychology*. New York: Springer.

Bunge, Silvia A. & Itamar Kahn. 2009. Cognition: Neuroimaging. In G. Adelman & B.H. Smith, eds. *Encyclopedia of Neuroscience*, Vol. 2, pp. 1063–1067. Amsterdam: Elsevier.

Cabieses, Fernando. 1993. *Apuntes de medicina tradicional*. Lima: Convenio Hipólito Unanue.

Canguilhem, Georges. 1966. *Le Normal et le Pathologique*. Paris: Presses Universitaires de France.

Carnap, Rudolf. 1950. *Logical Foundations of Probability*. Chicago: University of Chicago Press.

Charon, Rita. 2006. *Narrative Medicine: Honoring the Stories of Illness*. New York: Oxford University Press.

Cherkin, Daniel C. *et al.* 2009. A randomized trial comparing acupuncture, simulated acupuncture, and usual care for chronic low back pain. *Archives of Internal Medicine* 169: 858–866.

Chirac, Pierre & Els Torreele. 2006. Global framework on essential health R&D. *Lancet* 367: 1560–1561.

Cochrane Collaboration. 2013. Glossary. Retrieved from: www.cochrane.org

Collinger, Jennifer L., Brian Wodlinger, John E. Downey, Wei Yang. *et al.* 2013. High performance neuroprosthetic control by an individual with tetraplegia. *Lancet* 381: 557–564.

Cooter, Roger. 2007. After death/after "life": The social history of medicine in post-modernity. *Social History of Medicine* 20: 441–464.

D'Holbach, Paul-Henry Thiry, Baron. 1770. *Système de la nature*. 2 vols. Repr. Hildesheim: Georg Olms, 1966.

——. 1773. *Système social*. 2 vols. Repr. Hildesheim: Georg Olms, 1969.

Damasio, Antonio R. 1994. *Descartes' Error: Emotion, Reason, and the Human Brain*. New York: G.P. Putnam.

Dawes, Martin. *et al.* 2005. Sicily statement on evidence-based practice. *BMC Medical Education* 5: 11–18.

Dawes, Robyn M. 1996. *House of Cards: Psychology and Psychotherapy Built on Myth.* New York: Free Press.

Dawes, Robyn M., David Faust, & Paul E. Meehl. 1989. Clinical versus actuarial prediction. *Science* 243: 1668–1674.

Deary, Ian J. *et al.* 2012. Genetic contributions to stability and change in intelligence from childhood to old age. *Nature* 482: 212–215.

De Finetti, Bruno. 1972. *Probability, Induction, and Statistics.* New York: John Wiley & Sons.

De Smet, Peter A.G.M. 2002. Herbal remedies. *New England Journal of Medicine* 347: 2046–2056.

Diamond, Jared. 1997. *Guns, Germs, and Steel.* New York: W.W. Norton.

DiLorenzo, Daniel J. & Joseph D. Bronzino, eds. 2008. *Neuroengineering.* Boca Raton: CRC Press.

Dilthey, Wilhelm. 1883. *Introduction to the Human Sciences.* Princeton: Princeton University Press, 1989.

Dirac, Paul A.M. 1958. *The Principles of Quantum Mechanics.* 4th ed. Oxford: Clarendon Press.

Dreyfus, Stuart A. & Hubert L. Dreyfus. 1980. *A Five-Stage Model of the Mental Activities Involved in Directed Skill Acquisition.* Washington, DC: Storming Media.

Dubertret, Louis. 2006. Patient-based medicine. *Journal of the European Academy of Dermatology and Venereology* 20: 73–76.

Dubos, René. 1959. *The Mirage of Health.* New York: Praeger.

Duhem, Pierre. 1908. ΣΩΖΕΙΝ ΤΑ ΦΑΙΝΟΜΕΝΑ: *Essai sur la notion de théorie physique de Platon à Galilée.* Offprint from the *Revue de philosophie chrétienne.* Paris: Hermann.

Dworkin, Barry R. & Neal E. Miller. 1986. Failure to replicate visceral learning in acute curarized rat preparation. *Behavioral Neuroscience* 100: 299–314.

Eddy, Charles. 1982. Probabilistic reasoning in clinical medicine: Problems and opportunities. In D. Kahneman, P. Slovic, & A. Tversky, eds. *Judgment Under Uncertainty: Heuristics and Biases*, pp. 249–267. New York: Cambridge University Press.

Eddy, David M. & Charles H. Clanton. 1982. The art of diagnosis. *New England Journal of Medicine* 306: 1263–1268.

Einhorn, Hillel J. & Robin M. Hogarth. 1978. Confidence in judgment: Persistence of the illusion of validity. *Psychological Review* 85: 395–416.

Emanuel, Ezekiel. 2012. Prevention and cost control. *Science* 337: 1433.

Engels, Friedrich. 1883. *Dialectics of Nature*. New York: International Publishers, 1925.

Ezzati, Majid & Elio Riboli. 2012. Can noncommunicable diseases be prevented? Lessons from studies of populations and individuals. *Science* 337: 1482–1486.

Fisher, Ronald A. 1935. *The Design of Experiments*. 6th ed. London: Oliver and Boyd, 1951.

Fleck, Ludwik. 1935. *Genesis and Development of a Scientific Fact*. Preface by Thomas S. Kuhn. Chicago: University of Chicago Press, 1979.

Flexner, Abraham. 1910. *Medical Education in the United States and Canada: A Report to the Carnegie Foundation*. Boston: Updike.

Flier, Jeffrey S. 2013. Creating a Nobel culture. *Science* 339: 140–141.

Foddy, Bennett. 2009. A duty to deceive: Placebos in clinical practice. *American Journal of Bioethics* 9: 4–12.

Foucault, Michel. 1963. *Naissance de la clinique: Une archéologie du regard médical*. Paris: Presses Universitaires de France.

Freddi, Goffredo & José-Luis Román-Pumar. 2011. Evidence-based medicine: What it can and cannot do. *Annali dell'Istituto Superiore di Sanità* 47: 22–25.

Fuster, Joaquín M. 2006. The cognit: A network model of cortical representation. *International Journal of Psychophysiology* 60: 125–132.

Galilei, Galileo. 1623. *Il saggiatore*. In F. Flora, ed. *Opere [di G.G.]* Milano & Napoli: Ricciardi, 1953.

Gardner, Martin. 1957. *Fads and Fallacies*. New York: Dover.

Gibbons, Ann. 2012. An evolutionary theory of dentistry. *Science* 336: 973–975.

Gifford, Fred, ed. 2011. *Handbook of Philosophy of Science*, Vol. 16: *Philosophy of Medicine*. Amsterdam: Elsevier.

Gilbert, Bentley B. 1966. *The Evolution of National Insurance in Great Britain*. London: Joseph.

Gintis, Herbert, Samuel Bowles, Robert Boyd, & Ernst Fehr, eds. 2005. *Moral Sentiments and Material Interests*. Cambridge: MIT Press.

Glasziou, Paul. 2011. Foreword to Howick 2011.

Goldacre, Ben. 2010. *Bad Science: Quacks, Hacks, and Big Pharma Flacks*. London: Faber and Faber.

Graham, Loren R. 1981. *Between Science and Values*. New York: Columbia University Press.

Greenhalgh, Trish. 2012. Less research is needed. *Speaking of Medicine*, 14 August 2012.

Groopman, Jerome. 2008. *How Doctors Think*. Boston: Houghton Mifflin.

Groopman, Jerome & Paula Hartzband. 2011. *Your Medical Mind: How to Decide What Is Right for You*. New York: Penguin.

Grove, William M., David H. Zald, Boyd S. Lebow, Beth S. Snitz, & Chad Nelson. 2000. Clinical versus mechanical prediction: A meta-analysis. *Psychological Assessment* 12: 19–30.

Hacking, Ian. 1983. *Representing and Intervening*. Chicago: University of Chicago Press.

Hayward, Rodney A. & Harlan M. Krumholz. 2012. Three reasons to abandon low-density lipoprotein targets. *Circulation* 5: 2–5.

Hippocrates. 430–420 B.C. *Hippocrates Collected Works I*. W.H.S. Jones, ed. Cambridge: Harvard University Press; London: William Heinemann, 1948.

Howick, Jeremy. 2011. *The Philosophy of Evidence-Based Medicine*. Oxford: Wiley-Blackwell.

Howson, Colin & Peter Urbach. 1989. *Scientific Reasoning: The Bayesian Approach*. La Salle: Open Court.

Hume, David. 1710. *A Treatise of Human Nature*. Oxford: Clarendon Press, 1888.

Humphreys, Paul. 1985. Why propensities cannot be probabilities. *Philosophical Review* 94: 557–570.

Ioannidis, John P.A. 2005. Why most published research findings are false. *PLoS Medicine* 2(8): e124, doi: 10.1371/journal.pmed.0020124

Iversen, Leslie. 2001. *Drugs: A Very Short Introduction*. Oxford: Oxford University Press.

Jones, David, Scott H. Podolsky, & Jeremy A. Greene. 2012. The burden of disease and the changing task of medicine. *New England Journal of Medicine* doi: 10.1056/NEJMp1113569

Jones, Stephen R.G. 1992. Was there a Hawthorne effect? *American Journal of Sociology* 98: 451–466.

Kahneman, Daniel. 2011. *Thinking, Fast and Slow*. New York: Farrar, Straus and Giroux.

Kahneman, Daniel, Paul Slovic, & Amos Tversky, eds. 1982. *Judgment Under Uncertainty: Heuristics and Biases*. Cambridge: Cambridge University Press.

Kant, Immanuel. 1787. *Kritik der reinen Vernunft*. 2nd ed. (B). Hamburg: Felix Meiner, 1952.

Katzung, Bertram G., Susan B. Masters, & Anthony J. Trevor, eds. 2007. *Basic & Clinical Pharmacology*. 12th ed. Norwalk: Lange.

Kemeny, Margaret E. 2009. Psychobiological responses to social threat: Evolution of a psychological model in psychoneuroimmunology. *Brain, Behavior and Immunity* 23: 1–9.

Keyfitz, Nathan. 1984. Biology and demography. In N. Keyfitz, ed. *Population and Biology: Bridge Between Disciplines*, pp. 1–7. Liège: Ordina Editions.

Kim, Jaegwon. 2006. *Philosophy of Mind*. 2nd ed. Cambridge: Westview Press.

Kiple, Kenneth F., ed. 1993. *Cambridge World History of Human Diseases*. 2 vols. New York: Cambridge University Press.

Kirkup, Thomas. 1892. *History of Socialism*. London & Edinburgh: Adam and Charles Black.

Kirsch, Irving. 1985. Response expectancy as a determinant of experience and behavior. *American Psychologist* 40(11): 1189–1202.

Koepsell, David. 2009. *Who Owns You?* Malden: Wiley-Blackwell.

Kornberg, Arthur. 1989. *For the Love of Enzymes*. Cambridge: Harvard University Press.

Krikorian, Yervant H. 1944. *Naturalism and the Human Spirit*. Morningside Heights: Columbia University Press.

Kripke, Saul. 1971. Identity and necessity. In M.K. Munitz, ed. *Identity and Individuation*, pp. 135–164. New York: New York University Press.

Kupferschmidt, Kai. 2012. Uncertain verdict as vitamin D goes on trial. *Science* 337: 1476–1478.

Lane, Richard D. *et al.* 2009. The rebirth of neuroscience in psychosomatic medicine, Part II. *Psychosomatic Medicine* 71: 135–151.

Latour, Bruno. 1999. *Pandora's Hope: Essays on the Reality of Science Studies*. Cambridge: Harvard University Press.

Lazcano, Antonio. 2007. What is life? A brief historical overview. *Chemistry and Biodiversity* 4: 1–15.

Lewontin, Richard C. & Richard Levins. 2007. *Biology Under the Influence*. New York: Monthly Review Press.

Light, Donald & Joel Lexchin. 2012. Pharmaceutical research and development: What do we get for all that money? *British Medical Journal* 344: e4348.

Link, Bruce G. & Jo C. Phelan. 1995. Social conditions as fundamental causes of disease. *Journal of Health and Social Behavior* 35: 80–94.

Locke, John. [1690]. *An Essay Concerning Human Understanding.* New York: Dutton.

Locke, Steven E. & Mady Hornig-Rohan. 1983. *Mind and Immunity: Behavioral Immunology, an Annotated Bibliography.* Washington, DC: Institute for the Advancement of Health.

Longo, Dan, *et al.* 2011. *Harrison's Principles of Internal Medicine.* 2 vols., 18th ed. New York: McGraw-Hill.

Loscalzo, Joseph & Albert-Laszlo Barabasi. 2011. Systems biology and the future of medicine. *WIREs Systems Biology and Medicine* 3: 619–627.

Luisi, Pier Luigi. 2006. *The Emergence of Life: From Chemical Origins to Synthetic Biology.* Cambridge: Cambridge University Press.

McAlister, Alfred, Pekka Puska, & Jukka T. Salonen. 1981. Theory and action for health promotion: Illustrations from the North Karelia Project. *American Journal of Public Health* 72: 43–50.

McKeown, Thomas & Charles Ronald Lowe. 1967. *Introduction to Social Medicine.* Philadelphia: C.A. Davis Co.

Mackey, Allyson P., Kirstie J. Whitaker, & Silvia A. Bunge. 2012. Experience-dependent plasticity in white matter microstructure. *Frontiers in Neuroanatomy* 6: 1–8.

Mackey, Michael C. & Leon Glass. 1977. Oscillation and chaos in physiological control systems. *Science* 197: 287–297.

Mahner, Martin. 2012. The role of metaphysical naturalism in science. *Science and Education* 21(10): 1437–1459.

Mahner, Martin & Mario Bunge. 1997. *Foundations of Biophilosophy.* Berlin, Heidelberg, & New York: Springer.

Marmot, Michael G., Geoffrey Rose, Martin J. Shipley, & P.J. Hamilton. 1978. Employment grade and coronary heart disease in British civil servants. *Journal of Epidemiology and Community Health* 32: 244–249.

Marmot, Michael G., Jessica Allen, Ruth Bell, Ellen Bloomer, & Peter Goldblatt. 2012. WHO European review of social determinants of health and the health divide. *Lancet* 380: 1011–1029.

Mason, Stephen F. 1953. *A History of the Sciences.* London: Routledge & Kegan Paul.

Mata Pinzón, Soledad, ed. 2009. *Biblioteca Digital de la Medicina Tradicional Mexicana.*

Mattison, Julie A. *et al.* 2012. Impact of caloric restriction on health and survival in rhesus monkeys from the NIA study. *Nature* 489: 318–321.

Meehl, Paul E. 1954. *Clinical vs. Statistical Prediction: A Theoretical Analysis and a Review of the Evidence*. Minneapolis: University of Minnesota Press.

Merton, Robert K. 1973. *The Sociology of Science: Theoretical and Empirical Investigations*. Chicago: University of Chicago Press.

Merton, Robert K. & Elisa Barber. 2004. *The Travels and Adventures of Serendipity*. Princeton: Princeton University Press.

Mielczarek, Eugenie V. & Brian D. Engler. 2012. Measuring mythology. *Skeptical Inquirer* 36(1): 35–43.

Moonesinghe, Ramal, Muin J. Khoury, & A. Cecile J.W. Janssens. 2007. Most published research findings are false — but a little replication goes a long way. *PLoS Medicine* 4(2): e28: 0218–0221, doi: 10.371/journal.pmed.0040028

Mulet, José Miguel. 2011. *Los productos naturales ¡vaya timo!* Pamplona: Laetoli.

Murphy, Dominic. 2011. Conceptual foundations of biological psychiatry. In F. Gifford, ed. *Handbook of Philosophy of Science*, Vol. 16: *Philosophy of Medicine*, pp. 425–451. Amsterdam: Elsevier.

Murphy, Edmond A. 1997. *The Logic of Medicine*. 2nd ed. Baltimore, MD: Johns Hopkins University Press.

Nattrass, Nicoli. 2012. *The AIDS Conspiracy: Science Fights Back*. New York: Columbia University Press.

Nebert, Daniel W. & Ge Zhang. 2012. Personalized medicine: Temper your expectations. *Science* 337: 910.

Ness, Randolph M. & George C. Williams. 1994. *Why We Get Sick: The New Science of Darwinian Medicine*. New York: Vintage.

Nestler, Eric J. 2012. Stress makes its molecular mark. *Nature* 490: 171–174.

Nietzsche, Friedrich. 1886. *Beyond Good and Evil*. New York: Dover, 1997.

Ochsner, Kevin N. & James J. Gross. 2005. The cognitive control of emotion. *Trends in Cognitive Sciences* 9: 242–249.

Odling-Smee, John F., Kevin N. Laland, & Marcus W. Feldman. 2003. *Niche Construction*. Princeton: Princeton University Press.

Oparin, Alexander I. 1924. *The Origin of Life* [in Russian]. Moscow: Moscow Worker.

Osler, William. 1892. *The Principles and Practice of Medicine*. New York: Appleton.

Paracelsus. 1536. *Die große Wundartznei*. Ulm: Hans Varnier.

Park, Robert L. 2000. *Voodoo Science: The Road from Foolishness to Fraud*. New York: Oxford University Press.

Pascal, Blaise. 1963. *Oeuvres complètes*. Paris: Seuil.

Peña, Adolfo. 2010. The Dreyfus model of clinical problem-solving skills acquisition: A critical perspective. *Medical Education Online* 15, doi: 10.3402/meo.v15i0.4846

Perelson, Alan S. 2002. Modelling viral and immune system dynamics. *Nature Reviews* 2: 28–36.

Popper, Karl R. 1935. *The Logic of Scientific Discovery.* London: Heineman, 1958.

———. 1963. *Conjectures and Refutations.* London: Routledge & Kegan Paul.

Porter, Roy, ed. 1996. *Cambridge Illustrated History of Medicine.* Cambridge: Cambridge University Press.

———. 1997. *The Greatest Benefit to Mankind.* New York & London: W.W. Norton.

Ramachandran, Vilayanur S. 2011. *The Tell-Tale Brain.* New York: W.W. Norton.

Raz, Amir, Cory S. Harris, Veronica de Jong, & Hillel Braude. 2009. Is there a place for (deceptive) placebos within clinical practice? *American Journal of Bioethics* 9: 52–54.

Rigoutsos, Isidore & Gregory Stephanopoulos, eds. 2007. *Systems Biology.* Oxford: Oxford University Press.

Rizos, Evangelos C., Evangelia E. Ntzani, Eftychia Bika, Michael S. Kostapanos, & Moses S. Elisaf. 2012. Association between omega-3 fatty acid supplementation and cardiovascular disease events: A systematic review and analysis. *Journal of the American Medical Association* 308: 1024–1033.

Rosen, Gerald M. & Scott O. Lilienfeld. 2008. Posttraumatic stress disorder: An empirical evaluation of core assumptions. *Clinical Psychology Review* 28: 837–868.

Rosenhan, David L. 1973. On being sane in insane places. *Science* 179: 250–258.

Rubin, Donald B. 1974. Estimating causal effects of treatments in randomized and nonrandomized studies. *Journal of Educational Psychology* 66: 688–701.

Sackett, Davis L., William M.C. Rosenberg, J.A. Muir Gray, R. Brian Haynes, & W. Scott Richardson. 1996. Evidence based medicine: What it is and what it isn't. *British Medical Journal* 312: 71–72.

Sakurai, Masamoto. 2011. Herbal dangers. *Nature* 480: S97.

Sampson, Robert, J. 2012. Moving and the neighborhood glass ceiling. *Science* 337: 1464–1465.

Sanz, Victor-Javier. 2010. *La homeopatía ¡vaya timo!* Pamplona: Laetoli.

———. 2012. *La acupuntura ¡vaya timo!* Pamplona: Laetoli.

Saunders, Travis J., Mark S. Tremblay, Jean-Pierre Després, Claude Bouchard, Angelo Tremblay, & Jean-Philippe Chaput. 2013. Sedentary behavior, visceral fat accumulation and cardiometabolic risk in adults: A 6-year longitudinal study from the Quebec Family Study. *PLoS* 8: e54225.

Schwab, Martin E. & Anita Buchli. 2012. Plug the real brain drain. *Nature* 483: 267–268.

Sebreli, Juan José. 1992. *El asedio de la modernidad*. Barcelona: Ariel.

Shang, Aijing, Karin Huwiler-Müntener, Linda Nartey. *et al.* 2005. Are the clinical effects of homoeopathy placebo effects? Comparative study of placebo-controlled trials of homeopathy and allopathy. *Lancet* 366: 726–732.

Shelton, James D. 2013. Ensuring health in universal health coverage. *Nature* 493: 453.

Shook, John R. & Paul Kurtz, eds. 2009. *The Future of Naturalism*. Amherst, NY: Humanity Books.

Shorter, Edward. 1997. *A History of Psychiatry*. New York: John Wiley & Sons.

Shuchman, Miriam. 2005. *The Drug Trial: Nancy Olivieri and the Science Scandal that Rocked the Hospital for Sick Children*. Toronto: Random House.

Sigerist, Henry E. 1961. *A History of Medicine*, Vol. 2: *Early Greek, Hindu, and Persian Medicine*. Oxford: Oxford University Press.

Simon, Jeremy R. 2011. Medical ontology. In F. Gifford, ed. *Handbook of Philosophy of Science*, Vol. 16: *Philosophy of Medicine*, pp. 65–114. Amsterdam: Elsevier.

Singer, Charles. 1959. *A Short History of Scientific Ideas to 1900*. New York & London: Oxford University Press.

Skrabanek, Petr. 2000. *False Premises, False Promises*. Chippenham: Tarragon Press.

Sørensen, Per. *et al.* 2011. A randomized clinical trial of cognitive behavioural therapy versus short-term psychodynamic psychotherapy versus no therapy for patients with hypochondriasis. *Psychological Medicine* 41: 431–41.

Stuckler, David & Karen Siegler. 2011. *Sick Societies*. Oxford: Oxford University Press.

Tang, Jin-Ling, Si-Yan Zhan, & Edzard Ernst. 1999. Review of randomised controlled trials of traditional Chinese medicine. *British Medical Journal* 319: 160–161.

Taton, R[ené]. 1955. *Causalité et accidents de la recherche scientifique*. Paris: Masson.

Thomas, Lewis. 1983. *The Youngest Science: Notes of a Medicine-Watcher*. New York: Viking Press.

Thurler, Gerald. *et al.* 2003. Toward a systemic approach to disease. *ComPlexUs* 1: 117–122.

Tola, Fernando & Carmen Dragonetti. 2008. *Filosofía de la India*. Barcelona: Kairós.

Trigger, Bruce G. 2003. *Understanding Early Civilizations: A Comparative Study*. Cambridge: Cambridge University Press.

U.S. Department of Health and Human Services. 2012. Results from the 2011 National Survey on Drug Use and Health: Summary of national findings. Retrieved from www.samhsa.gov/data/nsduh/2k11results/nsduhresults2011.pdf

Urbach, Peter. 1985. Randomization and the design of experiments. *Philosophy of Science* 52: 256–273.

Valdizán, Hermilio. 1939. *Historia de la medicina peruana*. 3rd ed. Lima: Instituto Nacional de Cultura, 2005.

Van Fraassen, Bas C. 2008. *Scientific Representation: Paradoxes of Perspective*. Oxford: Clarendon Press.

Vane, John. 1971. Inhibition of prostaglandin synthesis as a machanism of action for aspirin-like drugs. *Nature* 231: 232–235.

Varma, Daya Ram. 2011. *The Art and Science of Healing Since Antiquity*. Bloomington: Xlibris.

Vaughan, Susan C., Randall D. Marshall, Roger D. McKinnon, Roger Vaughan, Lisa Mellman, & Steven P. Roose. 2000. Can we do psychoanalytic outcome research? *International Journal of Psychoanalysis* 81: 513–527.

Veatch, Robert M., ed. 1997. *Medical Ethics*. 2nd ed. Sudbury: Jones & Bartlett.

Vickers, Andrew J. 2012. Acupuncture for chronic pain: Individual patient data meta-analysis. *Archives of Internal Medicine* 172: 1444–1453.

Walter, Matthew. 2012. First, do harm. *Nature* 482: 148–152.

Wan, Poe Yu-Ze. 2011. *Reframing the Social: Emergentist Systemism and Social Theory*. Farnham: Ashgate.

Welch, H. Gilbert, Lisa M. Schwartz, & Steven Woloshin. 2011. *Overdiagnosed: Making People Sick in the Pursuit of Health*. Boston: Beacon Press.

White, Peter D., Hugh Rickards, & Adam Z.J. Zeman. 2012. Time to end the distinction between mental and neurological diseases. *British Medical Journal* 344: e3454.

White House. 2010. The necessity of science. Retrieved from: http://www.whitehouse.gov/blog/09/04/27

Wilkinson, Richard. 1992. Income distribution and life expectancy. *British Medical Journal* 304: 165–168.

Wilkinson, Richard & Kate Pickett. 2009. *The Spirit Level.* London: Penguin.

World Health Organization. 2011. *The World Medicines Situation 2011. Traditional Medicines: Global Situation, Issues and Challenges.* Geneva, Switzerland.

Worrall, John. 2002. What evidence in evidence-based medicine? *Philosophy of Science* 69: S316–S330.

———. 2007. Why there's no cause to randomize. *British Journal for the Philosophy of Science* 58: 451–488.

Wulff, Henrik R. 1981. *Rational Diagnosis and Treatment: An Introduction to Clinical Decision-Making.* 2nd ed. Oxford: Blackwell Scientific Publications.

Yong, Ed. 2012. Bad copy. *Nature* 485: 288–300.

Yudkin, John S., Kasia J. Lipska, & Victor M. Montori. 2011. The idolatry of the surrogate. *British Medical Journal* 343: d7795.

Zhang, Tie-Yuan & Michael J. Meaney. 2010. Epigenetics and the environmental regulation of the genome and its function. *Annual Review of Psychology* 61: 439–466.

PHILOSOPHICAL GLOSSARY

A

Axiology
Value theory.

B

Background knowledge
What is known so far, the starting point of a research project.

Bayesianism
Subjectivist interpretation of probability as credence or intensity of belief. Bayesians assign probabilities arbitrarily and do not believe in objective randomness.

C

Cause
Necessary and sufficient condition for something to happen.

Chance
Objective randomness or disorder.

Computationism
The programmatic hypothesis according to which natural or social processes of certain kinds (e.g., mental) are computational or algorithmic. Radical computationism holds that to be is to compute or to be computed.

Construct
Conceptual object: concept, proposition, norm, classification, or theory.

Constructivism
Ontological: The world is a human (individual or social) construction. *Epistemological*: All ideas are constructs, and none derive directly from perception.

Counter-Enlightenment
Reaction against the French Enlightenment. Targets: rationality, scientism, materialism, and democracy. Icons: Hegel, Nietzsche, and Heidegger.

Counterexample
Exception to an alleged law or rule. The popular saying "the exception that confirmed the rule" is absurd, for exceptions weaken generalizations.

D

Datum
A report on a fact, such as "She is sick." A scientific datum is one obtained with the help of a scientific technique, such as microscopy, and that can either confirm or infirm a hypothesis. Unlike facts, which are "hard," data can be more or less true.

Deontologism
The moral philosophy that binds us to duties regardless of consequences as well as to justice.

Determinism
Classical: Everything happens according to the laws of mechanics.
Modern: Everything happens according to laws, and nothing comes out of nothing.

Dialectics
The ontological doctrine, due to Hegel and adopted by Marx and his followers, according to which every item is at once the unity and struggle of opposites.

Dogmatism
Conceptual rigidity, refusal to face adverse facts and propose cogent arguments.
Antonym: Skepticism.

Dualism

The family of doctrines according to which there are two equally basic but mutually irreducible kinds, such as matter and mind, or nature and society. A particular case of pluralism.

E

Emergence

The advent of qualitative novelty. A property of systems. Examples: the emergence of AIDS and of AIDS therapies.
Synonym: Transcendence.

Empiricism

The epistemological doctrine according to which experience is the only source, content, and test of all ideas. Hippocrates and Hume were empiricists.

Energy

Changeability, the universal property of concrete things.

Enlightenment

The eighteenth-century cultural movement that exalted rationality, experience, the search for truth, utility, and solidarity.

Epistemology

The philosophical study of cognition and its product, knowledge. Main schools: skepticism, intuitionism, empiricism, conventionalism, fictionism, rationalism, ratioempiricism, and scientific realism.

Ethics

The philosophical study of morality, in particular moral norms, such as the Hippocratic Oath.

Event

Short-lasting change of a thing.

Evidence

A set of data relevant to some hypothesis.

Existence
The main property of an object. Conceptual existence: belonging to a conceptual system, such as a theory. Material existence: being a part of the real world, or having energy.

Experiment
Deliberate and controlled alteration of one or more properties of a thing, either to see what happens or to test a hypothesis.

Explanation
Description of a mechanism.

F

Fact
State or change of state of a material thing.

Functionalism
The view that only function matters, whereas "substrate" (matter) does not. The dominant view in contemporary philosophy of mind.

H

Hermeneutics
The school of thought according to which (a) symbols are all-important or even the only existents; and (b) all social facts are to be understood through the intuitive capture of the actors' intentions.

Holism
The family of doctrines according to which all things come in unanalyzable wholes. The ontological partner of intuitionism.
Antonym: Individualism.

Hypothesis
A proposition that asserts more than any data relevant to it. Example: psychoneural identity hypothesis.

I

Idealism, philosophical
The family of ontologies according to which ideas pre-exist and dominate everything else. Two main varieties: subjectivism (e.g., Berkeley and Kant) and objective realism (e.g., Plato and Hegel).

Indicator
Perceptible property or event that suggests an imperceptible trait or event. Example: the vital signs indicate the state of health.
Synonym: Marker.

Individualism
The view that the universe is an aggregate of separate individuals — that wholes and emergence are illusory.

Induction
The leap from a set of particular propositions to a universal proposition.

Inductivism
The thesis that all valid universal propositions are inductions.

Interdiscipline
A discipline formed by the fusion of two or more disciplines. Examples: biochemistry and cognitive neuroscience.

Intuition
Spontaneous (preanalytic) insight.

Intuitionism
The family of epistemological doctrines that asserts the primacy of intuition. The epistemological partner of holism.

L

Law
Regularity or pattern. Objective law: inherent in things, hence a property of theirs. Law statement: formula that captures an objective pattern. Sometimes called 'nomological statement' to avoid confusion with its referent.

Lawfulness, principle of
The philosophical hypothesis, presupposed in all the sciences, according to which everything, even chance, satisfies laws.

Level (of organization)
Collection of things characterized by a bundle of properties. Examples: physical, chemical, biological, social, semiotic, and technological levels.

Logic
The theory of deduction, inherent in all the disciplines.

M

Macro-reduction
Reduction to higher-level entities or processes. Example: explanation of individual facts in terms of her social standing.

Marker
See Indicator.

Material
Capable of changing by itself, having energy.

Materialism, philosophical
The family of naturalist ontologies according to which all existents are material. Three main versions: vulgar (or physicalist), dialectical, and emergentist (or systemic). Physicalism asserts that everything is physical. Dialectical (or Marxist) materialism is the fusion of materialism with dialectics: every existent is at once material and the unity of opposites. And emergentist (or systemic) materialism is the fusion of materialism with systemism: every existent is at once material and a system or part of one.

Matter
The set of all material things.

Meaning, semantic
A property of constructs. Reference or denotation together with sense or connotation. Not to be confused with the goal of an action.

Mechanism

The totality of processes that make a system tick, such as metabolism in the case of organisms, and healing in that of clinics.

Metaphysics

See Ontology.

Method, scientific

Background knowledge → Problem → Hypothesis or technique (special method) → Test → Evaluation → Revision of background knowledge → New problem. . .

Methodology

The part of epistemology that studies methods.

Micro-reduction

Reduction to lower-level entities. Examples: the growth and regeneration of tissues through cell division, and the attempt to explain everything social in biological terms.

Mind

Primitive view: The immaterial soul, or else the set of mental faculties or functions, that may be understood without the help of neuroscience. *Scientific view:* The family of specific functions of highly developed brains, whence it can only be explained by cognitive and affective neuroscience.

Mind-body problem

The question of the nature of the mental functions and their relation to the brain. Main answers:

(1) *Mysterianism* (Emil du Bois-Reymond, Colin McGinn, and Noam Chomsky): both matter and mind are and will always be unknowable;
(2) *Eliminative materialism* (e.g., Paul Churchland): there is only matter;
(3) *Radical spiritualism* (e.g., George Berkeley): there is no matter;
(4) *Moderate spiritualism* (e.g., Plato and John C. Eccles): the mind dominates the brain;
(5) *Parallelist dualism* (e.g., Spinoza): the cerebral and the mental processes are mutually independent but parallel;

(6) *Interactionist dualism* (e.g., Descartes, Freud, and Popper): the brain and matter are distinct but interacting entities;

(7) *Neutral monism* (e.g., Spencer and Feigl): there is a single unknowable entity, neither material nor mental, that looks material from the outside and ideal from the inside;

(8) *Psychoneural monism* (e.g., Hippocrates, Pinel, Cajal, and Hebb): mental processes are brain processes; and

(9) *Systemic psychoneural monism* (contemporary cognitive neuroscience and Bunge): psychoneural monism with the caveats that the brain interacts with other bodily organs as well as with the natural and social environments.

N

Naturalism
The family of ontologies that assert that all existents are natural — hence none are supernatural.

O

Objective
Referring to the object of study, not its student.
Synonym: Third-person account.

Objectivism
The thesis that it is possible and desirable to account for the external world in purely objective terms.

Ontology
The philosophical study of being and becoming.
Synonym: Metaphysics.

P

Phenomenalism
The philosophical view that there are only phenomena (appearances to someone), or that only these can be known. Phenomenalism is anthropocentric and it opposes realism.

Phenomenon
Perception of a fact, in contradistinction to the fact in itself. For instance, color as distinct from wavelength. Phenomena are real but they happen only in brains.

Plausibility
Consistency with the bulk of antecendent knowledge. Example: biologically plausible mechanism of the action of a drug.

Pluralism
The family of philosophies that assert the plurality of basic kinds (substance pluralism), basic properties (property pluralism), or both. Emergentist (or systemic) materialism is property-pluralist but substance-monist: one substance (matter), many properties.

Positivism
Modern empiricism. Classical positivism (Comte, Mill, Mach) was phenomenalist, inductivist, and diffident of theory. Logical positivism (Schlick, Carnap, Reichenbach) was phenomenalist, attempted to reduce the theoretical to the empirical, and stressed the importance of modern logic.

Postmodernism
The rejection of the intellectual values of the French Enlightenment, in particular clarity, consistency, and objective truth. A combination of hermeneutics with irrationalism.

Pragmatism
The philosophical doctrine according to which practice is the source, measure, and goal of all knowledge and all value.

Praxiology
Action theory.

Predicate
Conceptualization of a property. Predicates can be unary, like "is young"; binary, like "older than"; ternary, like "between"; and in general n-ary.

Primary/secondary quality
A primary quality or property is one that objects possess independently of their being perceived or acted on. Examples: acidity, dehydrated, and

infected. A secondary or subjective quality is subject-dependent. Examples: color, feeling unwell, and thirst.

Probability
Quantitative possibility.

Process
A non-instantaneous change of state of a thing: a sequence of states of a thing.

Property
Feature or trait of an item, such as the length of a segment, the energy of a bullet, the age of an organism, and the structure of a social group. There are neither properties without bearers, nor objects without properties.

Proposition
A statement, such as "You are reading," capable of being true or false to some degree. Any given statement can be expressed by a number of different sentences.

Pseudoscience
A body of belief or a practice sold as scientific although it is either untestable or at variance with the bulk of extant knowledge. Examples: homeopathy and psychoanalysis.

R

Ratioempiricism
Blend of rationalism and empiricism. Examples: Kant, logical empiricism, and scientific realism.

Rationalism
The epistemological doctrine according to which cognition involves reasoning. Radical or aprioristic rationalism: reason is sufficient for knowing. Moderate rationalism: reason is necessary for understanding.

Real
Existent in and by itself, that is, whether or not it is perceived or conceived by someone. Idealism holds that ideas are real; materialism that only material items are real.

Realism

The philosophy according to which the external world exists independently of the inquirer, and can be known at least in part. Scientific realism is the variety of idealism that takes scientific research to be the best means to acquire knowledge.

Reduction

Conceptual operation whereby an item is shown to be identical with another or included in it, or to be either an aggregate, a combination, or an average of other items.

Reductionism

Research strategy that attempts to understand complex things in terms of their composition.

Relativism

The opinion that there are no objective truths, that every idea is culture-bound.

Rule

Standardized prescription for doing something, or human behavior pattern. To be distinguished from 'law.' Example: a medical prescription.

S

Science

The branch of knowledge characterized by rationality, testability, and systemicity. Science is split into two great domains: formal (logic and mathematics), and factual-natural, biosocial, and social.

Scientism

The epistemological thesis that whatever can be known is investigated scientifically. Not to be confused with the disregard for non-physical features.

Sectarianism

Dogmatism combined with extremism.

Semantics

The study of meaning and truth. Not to be confused with 'a mere matter of words.'

Skepticism
The family of epistemologies that either deny the possibility of knowledge (radical or dogmatic skepticism), or else affirm that we should doubt and check before believing — and often even after having accepted a belief (moderate or methodological skepticism).

State (of a thing)
List of properties of a thing at a given instant.

State space
The set of all the possible states of a thing at a given instant. A state space has as many dimensions as the properties occurring in the states it represents.

Structure of a system
The totality of relations among the system's components, and among these and the system's environment.

Subjective
Something happening inside a subject's head, such as feeling thirsty or elated.

Subjectivism
The family of philosophies according to which everything is in a subject's mind (subjective idealism), or nothing can be known objectively.
Antonym: 'Objectivism.'

System
A complex object whose constituents are held together by strong bonds — logical, physical, biological, or social — and possessing global (emergent) properties that their parts lack.

Systemics
The branch of ontology concerned with the features common to all concrete systems.

Systemism
Ontology: Everything is either a system or a component of some system.
Epistemology: Every piece of knowledge is or ought to become a member of a conceptual system, such as a theory.

Axiology: Every value is or ought to become a component of a system of interrelated values.

T

Tautology
A truth of logic, such as "A or not-A," and "People rebound after being hurt because they are resilient."

Technology
Body of practical knowledge invented and utilized to design, produce, or maintain artifacts, whether physical (like computers), biological (like farm animals), or social (like clinics).

Testability, empirical
The ability of a hypothesis or a theory to be either confirmed or falsified to some extent by empirical data. A characteristic of science and scientific philosophy in contradistinction to theology and esotericism.

Theory
Hypothetico-deductive system: a system of propositions every one of which implies others or is implied by others. A well-organized (or axiomatized) theory is representable as an inverted branching bush starting with the assumptions (postulates and definitions) followed by their logical consequences.

Truth value
One of the various degrees of adequacy (true, false, half-true, etc.) that a proposition may have or acquire.

Truth, factual
The adequacy of an idea to the facts it represents, as with "it rains" while it is actually raining.

Truth, formal
The coherence of an idea with a previously accepted body of ideas. Examples: tautologies and theorems.

Truth, partial
The less-than-perfect adequacy of an idea to its referent, as in "$\pi = 3$."

U

Utilitarianism

The moral philosophy that enjoins us to maximize the expected utility or gain for self or others. Rivals: deontologism ("Do your duty regardless of consequences") and agathonism ("Seek the good for self or others").

Utility

Subjective value. For instance, placebo objects and recreational drugs.

V

Value, objective

The worth of something for the attainment of a goal, as in nutritive value. Not to be confused with desiratum, which may be subjective.

INDEX